Central Nervou Infections

D1583960

Editor

CYNTHIA BAUTISTA

CRITICAL CARE NURSING CLINICS OF NORTH AMERICA

www.ccnursing.theclinics.com

Consulting Editor
JAN FOSTER

September 2013 • Volume 25 • Number 3

BLOOMSBURY
HEALTHCARE LIBRARY
52 GOWER STREET
LONDON WC1E 6EB
0203-447-9097

ELSEVIER

1600 John F. Kennedy Boulevard • Suite 1800 • Philadelphia, Pennsylvania, 19103-2899

http://www.theclinics.com

CRITICAL CARE NURSING CLINICS OF NORTH AMERICA Volume 25, Number 3
September 2013 ISSN 0899-5885, ISBN-13: 978-0-323-18850-0

Editor: Katie Saunders
Developmental Editor: Donald Mumford

© **2013 Elsevier Inc. All rights reserved.**

This periodical and the individual contributions contained in it are protected under copyright by Elsevier, and the following terms and conditions apply to their use:

Photocopying

Single photocopies of single articles may be made for personal use as allowed by national copyright laws. Permission of the Publisher and payment of a fee is required for all other photocopying, including multiple or systematic copying, copying for advertising or promotional purposes, resale, and all forms of document delivery. Special rates are available for educational institutions that wish to make photocopies for non-profit educational classroom use. For information on how to seek permission visit www.elsevier.com/permissions or call: (+44) 1865 843830 (UK)/(+1) 215 239 3804 (USA).

Derivative Works

Subscribers may reproduce tables of contents or prepare lists of articles including abstracts for internal circulation within their institutions. Permission of the Publisher is required for resale or distribution outside the institution. Permission of the Publisher is required for all other derivative works, including compilations and translations (please consult www.elsevier.com/permissions).

Electronic Storage or Usage

Permission of the Publisher is required to store or use electronically any material contained in this periodical, including any article or part of an article (please consult www.elsevier.com/permissions). Except as outlined above, no part of this publication may be reproduced, stored in a retrieval system or transmitted in any form or by any means, electronic, mechanical, photocopying, recording or otherwise, without prior written permission of the Publisher.

Notice

No responsibility is assumed by the Publisher for any injury and/or damage to persons or property as a matter of products liability, negligence or otherwise, or from any use or operation of any methods, products, instructions or ideas contained in the material herein. Because of rapid advances in the medical sciences, in particular, independent verification of diagnoses and drug dosages should be made.

Although all advertising material is expected to conform to ethical (medical) standards, inclusion in this publication does not constitute a guarantee or endorsement of the quality or value of such product or of the claims made of it by its manufacturer.

Critical Care Nursing Clinics of North America (ISSN 0899-5885) is published quarterly by Elsevier Inc., 360 Park Avenue South, New York, NY 10010-1710. Months of issue are March, June, September, and December. Business and Editorial Offices: 1600 John F. Kennedy Blvd., Suite 1800, Philadelphia, PA 19103-2899. Periodicals postage paid at New York, NY and additional mailing offices. Subscription prices are $144.00 per year for US individuals, $308.00 per year for US institutions, $76.00 per year for US students and residents, $192.00 per year for Canadian individuals, $385.00 per year for Canadian institutions, $219.00 per year for international individuals, $385.00 per year for international institutions and $111.00 per year for Canadian and foreign students/residents. To receive student/resident rate, orders must be accompanied by name of affiliated institution, data of term, and the *signature* of program/residency coordinator on institution letterhead. Orders will be billed at individual rate until proof of status is received. Foreign air speed delivery is included in all *Clinics* subscription prices. All prices are subject to change without notice. **POSTMASTER:** Send address changes to *Critical Care Nursing Clinics of North America*, Elsevier Health Sciences Division, Subscription Customer Service, 3251 Riverport Lane, Maryland Heights, MO 63043. **Customer Service: 1-800-654-2452 (US and Canada); 314-447-8871 (outside US and Canada). Fax: 314-447-8029. E-mail: JournalsCustomerService-usa@elsevier.com (for print support) and JournalsOnlineSupport-usa@elsevier.com (for online support).**

Reprints. For copies of 100 or more of articles in this publication, please contact the Commercial Reprints Department, Elsevier Inc., 360 Park Avenue South, New York, New York, 10010-1710; Tel.: (212) 633-3813, Fax: (212) 462-1935, and E-mail: reprints@elsevier.com.

Critical Care Nursing Clinics of North America is covered in *MEDLINE/PubMed (Index Medicus)*, *International Nursing Index*, *Nursing Citation Index*, *Cumulative Index to Nursing and Allied Health Literature*, and *RNdex Top 100*.

Printed and bound by CPI Group (UK) Ltd, Croydon, CR0 4YY

Transferred to digital print 2012

Contributors

CONSULTING EDITOR

JAN FOSTER, PhD, RN, CNS
College of Nursing, Texas Woman's University, Houston, Texas

EDITOR

CYNTHIA BAUTISTA, PhD, RN, CNRN, CCNS, ACNS-BC
Neuroscience Clinical Nurse Specialist, Yale-New Haven Hospital, New Haven, Connecticut

AUTHORS

MARY MCKENNA GUANCI, MSN, RN, CNRN
Clinical Nurse Specialist, Neuroscience Intensive Care, Massachusetts General Hospital, Boston, Massachusetts

KATHERINE G. JOHNSON, MS, CNS-BC, CCRN, CNRN
Neuroscience Clinical Nurse Specialist, Patient Care Consulting Services, The Queens Medical Center, Honolulu, Hawaii

TESS SLAZINSKI, MN, RN, CCRN, CNRN, CCNS
Neuroscience Clinical Nurse Specialist, Critical Care Nursing Services, Cedars-Sinai Medical Center, Los Angeles, California

MISTI TUPPENY, MSN, CNS, CCRN, CNRN, CCNS
Neuroscience Clinical Nurse Specialist, Center for Nursing Education, Florida Hospital, Orlando, Florida

MICHELLE VANDEMARK, MSN, RN, ANP-BC
Clinical Instructor, Sanford School of Medicine, University of South Dakota, Sioux Falls, South Dakota

BLOOMSBURY HEALTHCARE LIBRARY
52 GOWER STREET
LONDON WC1E 6EB
0203-447-097

Contents

BLOOMSBURY
HEALTHCARE LIBRARY
52 GOWER STREET
LONDON WC1E 6EB
0203-447-9097

Preface: Central Nervous System Infections   ix

Cynthia Bautista

Acute Bacterial Meningitis: Current Review and Treatment Update   351

Michelle VanDemark

Bacterial meningitis is an infection of the meninges that can be infected by bacteria, virus, or fungus. The classic triad of bacterial meningitis consists of fever, neck stiffness, and altered mental status; headache is also another common symptom. Interventions for bacterial meningitis include prompt diagnosis, and initiation of antimicrobial therapy to optimize bacterial kill and decrease inflammatory response in the subarachnoid space. Nursing management consists of effective delivery of antibiotic therapy, fluid management, and supportive care.

Viral Meningitis and Encephalitis   363

Misti Tuppeny

Meningitis is an inflammation of the meninges, whereas encephalitis is inflammation of the parenchymal brain tissue. The single distinguishing element between the 2 diagnoses is the altered state of consciousness, focal deficits, and seizures found in encephalitis. Consequently meningoencephalitis is a term used when both findings are present in the patient. Viral meningitis is not necessarily reported as it is often underdiagnosed, whereas encephalitis cases are on the increase in various areas of North America. Improved imaging and viral diagnostics, as well as enhanced neurocritical care management, have improved patient outcomes to date.

Brain Abscess   381

Tess Slazinski

A brain abscess is defined as a localized collection of pus within the parenchyma of the brain or meninges. Brain abscesses are a complication of ear, sinus, and/or dental infections. Although they may occur in many brain locations, the most common sites are frontal and temporal lobes. Modern neuroimaging and laboratory analysis have led to prompt diagnosis and have decreased the mortality rates from brain abscess. Critical care nurses have a vital role in performing accurate neurologic assessments, timely administration of antibiotics, and management of fever.

Spinal Epidural Abscess   389

Katherine G. Johnson

Spinal epidural abscess is a rare bacterial infection located within the spinal canal. Early diagnosis and rapid treatment are important because of its potential to cause rapidly progressive spinal cord compression and irreversible paralysis. A staphylococcus bacterial infection is the cause in most cases. Treatment includes antibiotics and possible surgical drainage of the abscess. A favorable neurologic outcome correlates with the severity and duration of neurologic deficits before surgery and the timeliness of the chosen intervention. It is important for the critical care nurse to monitor the patient's neurologic status and provide appropriate interventions.

Ventriculitis of the Central Nervous System   399

Mary McKenna Guanci

An infection of the ventricular system of the brain is referred to as ventriculitis. The signs and symptoms of ventriculitis include the triad of altered mental status, fever, and headache, as seen in the patient with meningitis. Identifying the organism responsible is important in determining the cause and in planning a treatment strategy. Nurses have a pivotal role in the early identification and management of the patient with ventriculitis.

Index   407

CRITICAL CARE NURSING
CLINICS OF NORTH AMERICA

FORTHCOMING ISSUES

December 2013
Hematology
Melissa McLenon and Mary Lou Warren, *Editors*

March 2014
Age-Related Complications of Critical Illness
Sonya Hardin, RN, PhD, CCRN, *Editor*

RECENT ISSUES

June 2013
Summer Incidents and Accidents
Stephen D. Krau, PhD, RN, CNE, *Editor*

March 2013
Diabetes
Celia M. Levesque, RN, MSN, NP-C, *Editor*

December 2012
Winter Trauma
Margaret M. Ecklund, MS, RN, CCRN, ACNP-BC, *Editor*

BLOOMSBURY
HEALTHCARE LIBRARY
52 GOWER STREET
LONDOM WC1E 6EB
0203-447-.097

DOWNLOAD Free App!

Review Articles THE CLINICS

NOW AVAILABLE FOR YOUR iPhone and iPad

Preface

Central Nervous System Infections

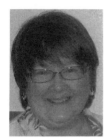

Cynthia Bautista, PhD, RN, CNRN, CCNS, ACNS-BC
Editor

The central nervous system (CNS) comprises the brain, spinal cord, and associated membranes. Viruses, bacteria, and fungi can infect the CNS. The clinical presentation will depend on the infecting agent and site of the infection. The following CNS infections will be presented in this issue that can be seen in the intensive care unit (ICU): ventriculitis, bacterial meningitis, viral meningitis, viral encephalitis, cerebral abscess, and spinal abscess. These conditions often require admission to an ICU or can be due to complications of ICU patients with a neurologic injury.

These CNS infections maybe encountered relatively infrequently in the ICU but they can cause morbidity and mortality for the ICU patient. CNS infections may have acute and chronic neurologic sequelae. Infections of the CNS can progress rapidly. An early diagnosis and timely initiation of appropriate antimicrobial therapy are the key goals of care for these patients. CNS infection patients can have an increased hospital length of stay and increased cost of hospital care and may necessitate further surgery.

The critical care nursing management of these patients with a CNS infection can be challenging. Critical care nurses need to be aware of the clinical features and treatment options for any ICU patient that might be experiencing a CNS infection. Having the knowledge to care for these patients is important to optimize their clinical outcome.

Cynthia Bautista, PhD, RN, CNRN, CCNS, ACNS-BC
Neuroscience Clinical Nurse Specialist
Yale-New Haven Hospital
New Haven, CT, USA

E-mail address:
cabbrain@aol.com

Crit Care Nurs Clin N Am 25 (2013) ix
http://dx.doi.org/10.1016/j.ccell.2013.04.006
0899-5885/13/$ – see front matter © 2013 Published by Elsevier Inc.

Acute Bacterial Meningitis
Current Review and Treatment Update

Michelle VanDemark, MSN, RN, ANP-BC

KEYWORDS

- Bacterial meningitis • Empiric antimicrobial therapy
- Adjunctive corticosteroids therapy • Petechial rash • Meningeal signs

KEY POINTS

- Acute bacterial meningitis is a life-threatening central nervous system (CNS) infection that requires prompt diagnosis and treatment.
- Bacterial meningitis is an infection of the meninges (dura mater, arachnoid, and pia mater) that cover and protect the brain and spinal cord.
- Ninety-five percent of persons with bacterial meningitis present with 2 of the following 4 symptoms: fever, nuchal rigidity, altered mental status, and headache.
- Do not delay initiation of empiric antibiotic therapy; antibiotics should be targeted to person's age, causative pathogen, local epidemiology trends, and patterns of drug resistance.
- Perform an immediate lumbar puncture without a prior computed tomography scan in persons without any risk factors for brain herniation. Risk factors include: age >60 years, altered level of consciousness, immune status, new-onset seizures, CNS disease, or focal neurologic deficits.
- Adjunctive dexamethasone therapy is associated with lower mortality, fewer neurologic sequelae, and fewer hearing deficits, and is recommended for children and adults living in developed countries with a low prevalence of human immunodeficiency virus.

INTRODUCTION

Acute bacterial meningitis is a life-threatening central nervous system (CNS) infection that requires prompt diagnosis and treatment. The incidence of bacterial meningitis has decreased with the widespread use of conjugate vaccines and advances in antimicrobial therapy. However, there continue to be high mortality rates with bacterial meningitis and significant long-term neurologic sequelae among survivors, especially in developing countries.[1–3] This review addresses the incidence, etiology, clinical features, diagnostic studies, and treatment of bacterial meningitis.

Neurocritical Care, Sanford USD Medical Center, 1305 West 18th Street, Sioux Falls, SD 57117-5039, USA
E-mail address: Michelle.vandemark@sanfordhealth.org

Crit Care Nurs Clin N Am 25 (2013) 351–361
http://dx.doi.org/10.1016/j.ccell.2013.04.004
0899-5885/13/$ – see front matter © 2013 Elsevier Inc. All rights reserved.

Bacterial meningitis is an infection of the meninges (dura mater, arachnoid, and pia mater) that cover and protect the brain and spinal cord. The meninges can be infected by bacteria, virus, or fungus. Bacterial meningitis may be a community-acquired or nosocomial infection. Nosocomial bacterial meningitis may result from a neurosurgical procedure such as a craniotomy, spinal surgery, lumbar drain, ventriculostomy, penetrating head trauma, or basal skull fractures.[4] The incidence of bacterial meningitis in the United States is approximately 1.3 to 1.9 cases per 100,000 persons annually.[2] In developing countries the incidence of bacterial meningitis is much higher, with approximately 2.6 to 6.0 cases per 100,000 persons annually.[5–8] There is a meningitis belt in Sub-Saharan Africa where several epidemics of meningococcal meningitis have occurred, and where the rates have exceeded 100 cases per 100,000 persons during an outbreak.[6,9]

EPIDEMIOLOGY

Common causative pathogens of bacterial meningitis include *Streptococcus pneumonia*, *Neisseria meningitides*, *Haemophilus influenzae*, group B streptococcus (GBS), *Listeria monocytogenes*, and *Streptococcus agalactiae*. The most common causative pathogens of bacterial meningitis are *S pneumonia* and *N meningitides*.[6,10] The epidemiology of bacterial meningitis has dramatically changed in the past few decades. In 1986, *H influenzae* was the leading cause of bacterial meningitis in the United States, accounting for approximately 45% of cases with the median age of 15 months.[6,11] With the introduction and widespread use of the *H influenzae* type b conjugate vaccine in infants and children in the 1990s, *H influenzae* infections have declined significantly, accounting for approximately 7% of cases of bacterial meningitis.[6] In 2007, the median age of persons with bacterial meningitis had increased to 41.9 years.[2] The heptavalent pneumococcal conjugate vaccine was introduced in the United States in 2000, and a tetravalent meningococcal conjugate vaccine was introduced in 2005. At present the leading cause of bacterial meningitis is *S pneumoniae*, accounting for approximately 60% of community-acquired meningitis.[2,6,10] Approximately 40% of persons with pneumococcal meningitis had a preceding sinusitis, otitis media, or respiratory infection.[6,10] The very young and the very old are most vulnerable for acquiring bacterial meningitis. Neonates younger than 2 months have an immature immune system and are still at high risk for developing bacterial meningitis, especially GBS.[2] Special risk groups such as neonates, the elderly, immunocompromised individuals, alcohol abusers, and pregnant women have a higher incidence of *L monocytogenes*.[11] Nosocomial infections following neurosurgical procedures are often caused by staphylococci, gram-negative bacilli, or anaerobic pathogens, resulting in bacterial meningitis.[12]

PATHOPHYSIOLOGY

The pathogenesis of bacterial meningitis begins with colonization of the nasopharyngeal mucosa or bacteremia from a systemic infection.[7,12] There are several different routes by which bacteria enter the CNS. First, bacteria can spread hematogenously and overcome the host defenses such as physical barriers, complement system, and blood-brain barrier, and invade the meninges. An alternative route is direct extension through emissary veins from a localized infection in the vicinity of the subarachnoid space such as sinusitis, otitis media, and mastoiditis. Finally, the bacteria can directly enter the subarachnoid space by way of a nosocomial infection following a neurosurgical procedure or a penetrating head wound.[12–14] The bacteria invade the meninges through the endothelium of choroid plexus and meningeal capillaries, resulting in hyperemia of blood vessels that increase the permeability of the blood-brain barrier.[8,15] Once past the blood-brain barrier, bacteria proliferate because the cerebrospinal fluid (CSF) contains low levels of immunoglobulins and complement components with which to combat an invasion, resulting in poor opsonization and phagocytosis. Replication and lysis of the bacteria trigger an inflammatory cascade in the CSF and subarachnoid space.[8] Meningeal inflammation develops, causing fever, meningismus, and altered mental status. Meningeal inflammation also increases the permeability of the blood-brain barrier, causing vasogenic edema.[9] The inflammation and breakdown of bacterial products can lead to neuronal injury resulting in hydrocephalus, vasculitis, abscess formation, and/or increased intracranial pressure (ICP) from cerebral edema.[8,12] Increased ICP can then cause decreased cerebral perfusion pressure and ischemia.[16]

The earlier the infection and inflammation is treated, the better the clinical outcome. When treatment is delayed bacteria can proliferate in the CSF, resulting in a higher density of bacterial-breakdown products and leading to increased inflammation. The cerebral damage results primarily from the immune response rather than the infection of the bacteria, so neurologic injury may continue even after the completion of antibiotic therapy.[8]

CLINICAL PRESENTATION

The clinical presentation of bacterial meningitis may range from an insidious progressive course over 3 to 5 days of malaise, fever, irritability, or vomiting, to a rapid fulminating course.[12] The classical triad of bacterial meningitis consists of fever, neck stiffness, and altered mental status; headache is also another common symptom. A prospective study of 696 adults with bacterial meningitis found that only 44% of cases presented with the classic triad, whereas 95% of cases presented with at least 2 of the 4 symptoms: fever, nuchal rigidity, altered mental status, and headache.[10] Fever is the most common and nonspecific symptom.[11] Meningeal irritation consists of headache, nuchal rigidity, and photophobia. The meningeal irritation can be demonstrated by the presence of a positive Kernig's sign or Brudzinski's sign. A positive Kernig's sign is produced by flexing both the hip and knee then extending the leg, which elicits pain in the hamstrings. A positive Brudzinski's sign is produced when the person is supine and the neck is passively flexed, resulting in involuntary flexion of the legs.[11] A meta-analysis of prospective studies found that neck stiffness was 51% sensitive, the Kernig's sign was 53% sensitive, and the Brudzinski's sign was 66% sensitive for the diagnosis of bacterial meningitis in children.[6,17] In adults, these diagnostic tests have less sensitivity.[6,18] A petechial rash can appear as tiny red or purple dots early in the course of a meningococcal infection. This rash can then progress to nonblanching purpural blotches in 90% of children and 60% of adults with N meningitides.[6] The petechial rash can develop under elastic waist bands or stockings, or in dependent areas such as the back of a supine person.[7] Other symptoms of bacterial meningitis may include aphasia, lethargy, malaise, vomiting, focal neurologic deficits, ataxia, and seizures.[10]

Neonates and infants may not present with the classic findings of bacterial meningitis, and instead may present with vague nonspecific symptoms such as a high-pitched or moaning cry, fever, lethargy, irritability, poor feeding, vomiting, diarrhea, respiratory distress, seizures, and bulging fontanels.[14,19] These vague symptoms make the diagnosis of meningitis challenging. In addition, health care providers should consider the diagnosis of bacterial meningitis in any immunocompromised individual who presents with an infectious disease and a decrease in mental status.[14,16,20]

DIAGNOSIS

Diagnosis of bacterial meningitis begins with a complete medical history and comprehensive physical examination. During the medical history one must inquire about the person's recent illnesses, travel history, vaccinations, immunosuppressed conditions, illicit drug use, or exposure to persons with bacterial meningitis. However, the medical history and physical examination are not always sufficient to diagnose bacterial meningitis; a lumbar puncture for CSF analysis is necessary for a definitive diagnosis. Blood cultures should be drawn immediately. Blood cultures identify the causative organism in 50% to 80% of cases of bacterial meningitis, and should be obtained before the initiation of antimicrobial therapy. If the person was pretreated with antibiotics, the yield of blood cultures decreases by 20%.[6,21] Controversy exists regarding whether a computed tomography (CT) scan of the brain should be performed before a lumbar puncture. A CT scan of the brain would determine if the person has cerebral edema. Cerebral edema can increase the risk of brain herniation during a lumbar puncture. The Infectious Diseases Society of America (IDSA) recommends proceeding to immediate lumbar puncture without a prior CT scan in persons without any of the following risk factors: age greater than 60 years; altered level of consciousness or immunocompromised state (human immunodeficiency virus [HIV]/AIDS, posttransplant, receiving immunosuppressive therapy, asplenia, cancer); new-onset seizures (within 1 week); history of CNS disease (brain lesion, stroke, or focal infection); focal neurologic deficits such as papilledema, dilated nonreactive pupil, gaze, or facial palsy; abnormal language; inability to answer 2 questions or follow 2 commands; visual field abnormalities; and arm or leg drift (**Box 1**).[11,20,22,23] People identified as high risk for a lumbar puncture should have blood cultures and initiation of empiric antibiotic therapy before undergoing a CT scan. In the absence of any of these findings, blood cultures and a lumbar puncture should be immediately performed, followed by administration of empiric antibiotic therapy.[22]

Lumbar puncture provides for CSF analysis that identifies the organism and its susceptibility to various antibiotics. Ideally the lumbar puncture should be performed before initiation of antimicrobial therapy to maximize the yield of cultures.[7] Studies have found that complete sterilization of the CSF can occur within 2 to 4 hours after initiating antibiotics.[7,19,24] Analysis of the CSF is the gold standard, essential for the diagnosis of bacterial meningitis by identifying the causative organism and

---

Box 1
Clinical conditions that predict the need for head CT prior to a lumbar puncture when diagnosing bacterial meningitis

- Age > 60 years
- Altered level of consciousness
- Immunocompromised state (HIV/AIDS, immunosuppressive therapy, transplant recipient)
- History of CNS disease: brain lesion, stroke or focal infection
- New-onset seizures in past week
- Focal neurologic deficits such as papilledema, dilated pupil or visual field abnormalities
- Abnormal language
- Arm or leg drift inability of answer 2 questions or follow 2 commands

Data from Refs.[6,7,22,23]

susceptibility to antimicrobial therapy. CSF Gram stain was found to be positive for bacterial meningitis in 60% to 80% of cases, with yield decreasing to 7% to 41% among persons pretreated with antibiotics.[6,11,22] If the CSF specimen is obtained before antibiotics are started, the CSF culture is positive in 80% to 90% of cases and is diagnostic for bacterial meningitis; however, a time frame up to 48 hours may be needed for organism identification (**Fig. 1**).[6]

In bacterial meningitis the opening pressure of the lumbar puncture is elevated, greater than 180 mm H_2O. The CSF analysis predictive of bacterial meningitis includes: white blood cell (WBC; leukocyte) count greater than 2000 cells/mm^3 or CSF neutrophil count of more than 1180 cells/mm^3; protein concentration of more than 220 mg/dL; or a CSF glucose concentration of less than 34 mg/dL and a CSF-to-serum glucose ratio of less than 0.23.[6,10,22] Additional CSF studies that aid in the diagnosis include the latex agglutination antigen test and real-time polymerase chain reaction (PCR). Real-time PCR amplifies DNA to detect the presence of bacteria. Latex agglutination and real-time PCR tests may be especially helpful if lumbar puncture has been delayed and antimicrobial therapy initiated. CSF lactate concentration has been found to be more than 90% sensitive and specific in differentiating bacterial from aseptic meningitis. If antibiotics are administered before the lumbar puncture, the sensitivity of CSF lactate concentration decreases to 49%, limiting the usefulness of this test.[6,25] In addition, elevated C-reactive protein ($\geq$20 mg/L) and serum procalcitonin ($\geq$0.5 µg/L) concentrations are associated with bacterial meningitis rather than aseptic meningitis.[6,11,22]

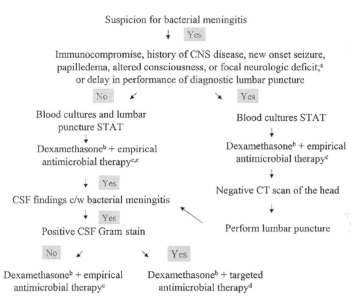

Fig. 1. Diagnostic algorithm for acute bacterial meningitis. [a] Includes those associated with CSF shunts, hydrocephalus, or trauma, those occurring after neurosurgery, or various space-occupying lesions. [b] Palsy of cranial nerve VI or VII is not an indication to delay lumbar puncture. [c] See text for recommendations for use of adjunctive dexamethasone in infants and children with bacterial meningitis. [d] See **Table 1**. [e] Dexamethasone and antimicrobial therapy should be administered immediately after CSF is obtained. (*From* Tunkel AR, Hart BJ, Kaplan SL, et al. Practice guidelines for the management of bacterial meningitis. Clin Infect Dis 2004;39:1270; with permission.)

TREATMENT

Strategies used to improve clinical outcomes from bacterial meningitis include prompt diagnosis of bacterial meningitis, and initiation of antimicrobial therapy to optimize bacterial kill and decrease the inflammatory response in the subarachnoid space.[5] Persons who present to the emergency department (ED) with a suspicion of bacterial meningitis should receive empiric broad-spectrum antibiotics immediately until the causative organism is identified. When selecting the most effective empiric antibiotics, consideration should be made regarding the most likely causative organism as well as the person's age, risk factors, immune status, setting of acquisition (community-acquired vs nosocomial), and local epidemiology.[3,6,22] If there is a delay in lumbar puncture, antibiotic therapy should be promptly initiated. A retrospective study by Proulx and colleagues[26] found that if antibiotics are initiated within 6 hours of presentation to the ED for a person with suspected bacterial meningitis, the case fatality rate is 5% to 6%. If antibiotic therapy is initiated 6 to 8 hours after arrival the case fatality rate increases to 45%, and if therapy starts 8 to 10 hours after arrival the case fatality rate increases to 75%.[7] Antimicrobial therapy for meningitis requires higher doses to penetrate the blood-brain barrier and be metabolized in the CSF.[1] Recommendations by the IDSA for empiric antibiotic therapy may include third-generation cephalosporins such as cefotaxime or ceftriaxone, plus penicillin G or ampicillin, plus vancomycin (**Table 1**). Third-generation cephalosporins have excellent CSF penetration and provide coverage for the most common bacterial pathogens, including *S pneumonia* and *N meningitis*.[11] Penicillin G and ampicillin have been shown to be effective against multiple bacterial pathogens and should be included in the empiric therapy, especially when *L monocytogenes* meningitis is suspected.[1,11,22] Vancomycin should be added to the therapeutic regime owing to concern for drug-resistant pathogens.[1] The global emergence of antibiotic-resistant pathogens and the slow development of new antibiotics have made bacterial meningitis an evolving therapeutic challenge.[3] After the results of the Gram stain, culture, and susceptibility have become available, and the causative pathogen has been identified, antibiotic therapy should be de-escalated.

The IDSA guidelines recommend the use of adjunctive dexamethasone in children or adults with suspected community-acquired bacterial meningitis.[22] Corticosteroids

Table 1		
Empiric antimicrobial therapy based on age and causative pathogen		
Age	**Common Bacterial Pathogens**	**Antimicrobial Therapy**
<1 mo	*Streptococcus agalactiae, Escherichia coli, Listeria monocytogenes, Klebsiella* spp	Ampicillin plus cefotaxime or ampicillin plus an aminoglycoside
1–23 mo	*Streptococcus pneumoniae, Neisseria meningitidis, S agalactiae, Haemophilus influenzae, E coli*	Vancomycin plus a third-generation cephalosporin[a,b]
2–50 y	*N meningitidis, S pneumoniae*	Vancomycin plus a third-generation cephalosporin[a,b]
>50 y	*S pneumoniae, N meningitidis, L monocytogenes*, aerobic gram-negative bacilli	Vancomycin plus ampicillin plus a third-generation cephalosporin[a,b]

[a] Ceftriaxone or cefotaxime.
[b] Some experts would add rifampin if dexamethasone is also given.
From van de Beek D, Brouwer MC, Thwaites GE, et al. Advances in treatment of bacterial meningitis. Lancet 2012;380:1694; with permission.

act to decrease the inflammation of the subarachnoid space caused by the bacterial products responsible for neuronal injury. Moreover, corticosteroids have been shown to stabilize the blood-brain barrier and reduce CSF outflow resistance, resulting in decreased ICP. Dexamethasone is the corticosteroid most often recommended for use in bacterial meningitis because of its ability to penetrate the CSF.[8] Reports exist regarding administration of adjunctive dexamethasone to reduce hearing loss in children with *H influenzae* type b meningitis.[6] In 2010, a Cochrane meta-analysis showed that use of adjunctive dexamethasone in children decreased the incidence of hearing loss but did not affect mortality.[6] The IDSA guidelines advise the administration of adjunctive dexamethasone before or with the first dose of antibiotics with continuance every 6 hours for 4 days. However, dexamethasone reduces the permeability of the blood-brain barrier, decreasing the clinical efficacy of large-molecule antimicrobials such as vancomycin in penetrating the CSF and thus delaying CSF sterilization.[1,3,22,27] Multiple studies have demonstrated conflicting results as to whether adjunctive dexamethasone is beneficial in adults with suspected community-acquired bacterial meningitis.[6] A European controlled trial showed that adjunctive dexamethasone was associated with a favorable outcome, resulting in fewer neurologic sequelae and a lower mortality rate among people with pneumococcal meningitis.[28] The European Dexamethasone in Adulthood Bacterial Meningitis Study showed that dexamethasone can provide extended survival benefits of up to 20 years in persons with bacterial meningitis.[29] However, a meta-analysis of more than 2000 persons with bacterial meningitis showed that adjunctive dexamethasone treatment did not reduce neurologic sequelae or decrease mortality.[30] These studies suggest that dexamethasone treatment is associated with lower mortality, fewer neurologic sequelae, and fewer hearing deficits in children and adults with pneumococcal meningitis who live in developed countries.[27] Adjunctive dexamethasone therapy is most efficacious for persons with community-acquired bacterial meningitis living in developed countries with a low HIV prevalence, whereas there may be no benefit for persons living in developing countries where the disease burden is highest and there is a high HIV prevalence, making dexamethasone ineffective.[6,8,31]

Nursing Management

Nursing management consists of effective delivery of antibiotic therapy, fluid management, and supportive care. Persons with bacterial meningitis should be placed on droplet isolation precautions until the organism has been identified and they have completed 24 hours of appropriate antibiotic therapy.[32] The neurologic status of patients with bacterial meningitis should be monitored closely, being alert for signs of increased ICP, altered level of consciousness, or seizures. Nursing responsibilities include airway protection, oxygenation monitoring, and administration of supplemental oxygen as needed. The temperature of patients should be monitored and treated aggressively with antipyretic agents, fans, and cooling measures. Fluid balance and electrolytes should be closely watched and treated as needed. A quiet darkened room to limit stimulation is recommended. Supportive care should be provided for persons with bacterial meningitis and their family.

PREVENTION

Chemoprophylaxis should be given to individuals who have had close contact with a person with *N meningitidis* or *H influenzae* type b meningitis within 1 week before the onset of symptoms.[16] Bacterial meningitis is caused by spread of the organism through water droplets from person to person, by intimate personal contact such as through kissing or sneezing, or close contact with an infected person. *N meningitidis* is a large droplet that may be transmitted easily through respiratory secretions or saliva. Persons at risk for acquiring *N meningitidis* include household members, intimate contacts, active or passive smokers, and/or living in crowded environments such as dormitories, military barracks, and child care centers.[7] Chemoprophylaxis includes antibiotics that reduce nasopharyngeal colonization including rifampin, ciprofloxacin, or ceftriaxone.[16]

Vaccinations provide the best protection against bacterial meningitis. Vaccines are available to protect against 3 common forms: *H influenzae* type b conjugate vaccine, heptavalent pneumococcal conjugate vaccine PCV7, and tetravalent meningococcal conjugate vaccine. Many of the current vaccines for bacterial meningitis do not protect against all forms of bacterial serotypes, creating a challenge when combating meningitis worldwide. Up to 90% of children in developed countries are protected by PCV7, but only 50% to 65% of children in developing countries.[33] However, the PCV7 does not cover all of the serotypes of pneumococcal disease. The meningococcal conjugate vaccine protects against serogroups A, C, W-135, and Y, which account for the majority of meningococcal disease. However, the vaccine does not cover serogroup B, which accounts for one-third of meningococcal disease.[12] Unfortunately, only 45% of the world's children have been fully immunized. Effort is needed to promote immunization programs worldwide, especially in developing countries.[33] The development of a universal vaccine with broad protection against pneumococcal and meningococcal meningitis serotypes would be a great benefit for the world's health.

OUTCOME

The incidence of bacterial meningitis has decreased in the past few decades primarily because of widespread vaccine use and improved antimicrobial therapy. The person's level of consciousness and the severity of the disease at presentation, plus the timeliness of antibiotic therapy, affect the prognosis of bacterial meningitis.[12] Several retrospective studies have identified risk factors associated with poor prognosis, including the causative organism, person's age greater than 60 years, comorbidities, presence of otitis media or sinusitis, low Glasgow Coma Scale score on admission, focal neurologic deficits, tachycardia, positive blood culture, absence of rash, elevated erythrocyte sedimentation rate, thrombocytopenia, and low CSF WBC count.[10,12] Worsened clinical outcomes are associated with tachycardia, hypotension, seizures, altered mental status, and CSF WBC count less than 1000 (**Box 2**).[11] The incidence of bacterial meningitis in older adults has remained high, and mortality increases with increasing age. In the United States, adults 18 to 34 years old had 8.9% mortality rate, whereas mortality rate was 22.7% in adults 65 years and older.[2] In developing countries, the mortality rate in adults with bacterial meningitis is 6% to 37% of cases.[2,6,27]

Neurologic sequelae occur in up to 50% of survivors following bacterial meningitis, and include hearing loss, seizures, hydrocephalus, developmental disorders, and neuropsychological impairment.[5,10] Permanent sensorineural hearing loss occurs in 5% to 35% of survivors of bacterial meningitis.[14] Approximately 27% of persons with pneumococcal meningitis suffer from neuropsychological sequelae.[27,30] Systemic complications in approximately 44% of survivors include hyponatremia, septic shock, adult respiratory distress syndrome, and disseminated intravascular coagulation.[14]

Bacterial meningitis remains a devastating disease, with significant morbidity and mortality especially in the very young and very old. Bacterial meningitis is an evolving

---

Box 2
Acute bacterial meningitis: indicators of poor prognosis

- Causative organism
- Age greater than 60 years old
- Comorbidities
- Altered mental status
- Low Glasgow Coma Scale score on admission
- Focal neurologic deficits
- Cerebrospinal fluid white blood cell count less than 1000
- Elevated erythrocyte sedimentation rate and thrombocytopenia
- Tachycardia and hypotension
- Seizures

Data from Refs.[10–12]

---

therapeutic challenge with the global emergence of multidrug-resistant pathogens. Empiric antibiotics should be administered promptly and be targeted to the person's age, causative organism, local epidemiology trends, and drug-resistance patterns. Diagnostic studies should be promptly and efficiently performed. A CT scan of the head should be done if the person has a decreased level of consciousness, focal neurologic deficits, or signs of increased ICP. CSF examination is crucial for the diagnosis of bacterial meningitis and identification of the causative organism. Medical treatment remains a challenge with the changing epidemiology of bacterial meningitis and the emergence of antimicrobial-resistant pathogens. Worldwide prevention measures and increased availability of vaccines, especially in developing countries, will aid in eliminating this devastating disease.

REFERENCES

1. Miranda J, Tunkel AR. Strategies and new developments in the management of bacterial meningitis. Infect Dis Clin North Am 2009;23:925–43.
2. Thigpen MC, Whitney CG, Messonnier NE, et al. Bacterial meningitis in the United States, 1998-2007. N Engl J Med 2011;364:2016–25.
3. van de Beek D, Brouwer MC, Thwaites GE, et al. Advances in treatment of bacterial meningitis. Lancet 2012;380:1693–702.
4. van de Beek D, Drake J, Tunkel AR. Nosocomial bacterial meningitis. N Engl J Med 2010;362:146–54.
5. van de Beek D, de Gans J, Tunkel AR, et al. Community-acquired bacterial meningitis in adults. N Engl J Med 2006;354:44–53.
6. Brouwer MC, Tunkel AR, van de Beek D. Epidemiology, diagnosis, and antimicrobial treatment of acute bacterial meningitis. Clin Microbiol Rev 2010;23:467–92.
7. Bhimraj A. Acute community-acquired bacterial meningitis in adults: an evidence based review. Cleve Clin J Med 2012;79:393–400.
8. Prasad K, Rai NK, Kumar A. Use of corticosteroids and other adjunct therapies for acute bacterial meningitis in adults. Curr Infect Dis Rep 2012;14:445–53.
9. Agrawal S, Nadel S. Acute bacterial meningitis in infants and children: epidemiology and management. Paediatr Drugs 2011;13:385–400.

10. van de Beek D, de Gans J, Spanjaard L, et al. Clinical features and prognostic factors in adults with bacterial meningitis. N Engl J Med 2004;351:1849–59.
11. Fitch MT, Abrahamian FM, Moran GJ, et al. Emergency department management of meningitis and encephalitis. Infect Dis Clin North Am 2008;22:33–52.
12. Roos KL, Greenlee JE. Meningitis and encephalitis. Neurology 2011;17:1010–23.
13. Koedel U, Klein M, Pfister HW. New understanding of the pathophysiology of bacterial meningitis. Curr Opin Infect Dis 2010;23:217–23.
14. Lin AL, Safdieh JE. The evaluation and management of bacterial meningitis: current practice and emerging developments. Neurologist 2010;16:143–51.
15. Gerber J, Nau R. Mechanisms of injury in bacterial meningitis. Curr Opin Neurol 2010;23:312–8.
16. Somand D, Meurer W. Central nervous system infections. Emerg Med Clin North Am 2009;27:89–100.
17. Curtis S, Stobart K, Vandermeer B, et al. Clinical features suggestive of meningitis in children: a systematic review of prospective data. Pediatrics 2010;126: 952–60.
18. Thomas KE, Hasbun R, Jekel J, et al. The diagnostic accuracy of Kernig's sign, Brudzinski's sign, and nuchal rigidity in adults with suspected meningitis. Clin Infect Dis 2002;35:46–52.
19. Kim KS. Acute bacterial meningitis in infants and children. Lancet Infect Dis 2010; 10:32–42.
20. Ziai WC, Lewin JJ. Update in the diagnosis and management of central nervous system infections. Neurol Clin 2008;26:427–68.
21. Nigrovic LE, Mallery R, Macias CG, et al. Effect of antibiotic pretreatment on cerebrospinal fluid profiles of children with bacterial meningitis. Pediatrics 2008; 122:726–30.
22. Tunkel AR, Hart BJ, Kaplan SL, et al. Practice guidelines for the management of bacterial meningitis. Clin Infect Dis 2004;39:1267–84.
23. Hasbun R, Abrahams J, Jekel J, et al. Computed tomography of the head before lumbar puncture in adults with suspected meningitis. N Engl J Med 2001;345: 1727–33.
24. Kanegaye JT, Soliemanzadeh P, Bradley JS. Lumbar puncture in pediatric bacterial meningitis: defining the time interval for recovery of cerebrospinal fluid pathogens after parenteral antibiotic pretreatment. Pediatrics 2001;108:1169–74.
25. Sakushima K, Hayashino Y, Kawaguchi T, et al. Diagnostic accuracy of cerebrospinal fluid lactate for differentiating bacterial meningitis from aseptic meningitis: a meta-analysis. J Infect 2011;62:255–62.
26. Proulx N, Fréchette D, Toye B, et al. Delays in the administration of antibiotics are associated with mortality from adult acute bacterial meningitis. QJM 2005;98: 291–8.
27. Borchorst S, Moller S. The role of dexamethasone in the treatment of bacterial meningitis—a systematic review. Acta Anaesthesiol Scand 2012;56(10):1210–21.
28. de Gans J, van de Beek D. Dexamethasone in adults with bacterial meningitis. N Engl J Med 2002;347:1549–56.
29. Fritz D, Brouwer MC, van de Beek D. Dexamethasone and long-term survival in bacterial meningitis. Neurology 2012;79:1–3.
30. van de Beek D, Farrar JJ, de Gans J. Adjunctive dexamethasone in bacterial meningitis: a meta-analysis of individual patient data. Lancet Neurol 2010;9: 254–63.
31. Cooper DD, Seupaul RA. Is adjunctive dexamethasone beneficial in patients with bacterial Meningitis? Ann Emerg Med 2012;59:225–6.

32. Siegel JD, Rhinehart E, Jackson M, et al, and the Healthcare Infection Control Practices Advisory Committee, 2007 Guideline for Isolation Precautions: Preventing Transmission of Infectious Agents in Healthcare Settings, June 2007. http://www.cdc.gov/ncidod/dhqp/pdf/isolation2007.pdf.
33. Bottomley MJ, Serruto K, Safadi MA, et al. Future challenges in the elimination of bacterial meningitis. Vaccine 2012;30(Suppl 2):B78–86.

Viral Meningitis and Encephalitis

Misti Tuppeny, MSN, CNS, CCRN, CNRN, CCNS

KEYWORDS

- Meningitis • Encephalitis • Meningoencephalitis • Central nervous system infections
- Viral infections • Brain infection

KEY POINTS

- Meningitis and encephalitis can be caused by a variety of commonly noted viruses or can spread via specific vectors with seasonal variability.
- The commonly noted signs and symptoms of viral meningitis or encephalitis are headache, fever, nuchal rigidity, focal deficits, or outright alteration in level of consciousness specific to encephalitis.
- Diagnostic workup is imperative in determining the specific viral syndrome and organism. The workup can include serology, specifically polymerase chain reaction (which aids in determining the specific viral antigen), radiologic tests, and lumbar puncture.
- Seasonal distribution and public health education is noted with viral encephalitis syndromes. The public must have an awareness of the specifics that can aid in the spread of encephalitis, and its impact on public health.

MENINGITIS

Viruses are the major cause of meningitis and are often underdiagnosed and, thus, not reported. **Table 1** identifies the various viral infections that can affect the central nervous system (CNS). The classification of viruses is divided according to whether the virus contains RNA or DNA.

Meningitis can occur in individuals of any age group, and is usually a self-limiting process characterized by signs of meningeal irritation (headache, photophobia, and nuchal rigidity). The term aseptic refers to the fact that the infection of the subarachnoid space and meninges has no bacterial organism that can be isolated or identified. If a specific virus can be identified, a physician is justified in using the term in diagnosing viral meningitis. However, owing to a myriad of factors (pathophysiology of multiple viral infections, lack of interest in diagnosing a non–life-threatening syndrome, lack of accessibility, and expense of viral isolation procedures), the diagnosis often rests primarily on clinical grounds, which only then is substantiated by serologic

Disclosures: The author has no financial disclosures or conflicts of interest.
Center for Nursing Education, Florida Hospital, 601 East Rollins Avenue, Orlando, FL 32803, USA
E-mail address: misti.tuppeny@flhosp.org

Table 1
Viral infection of the nervous system

Virus Type	Representative Viruses Responsible for Neurologic Disease
RNA Viruses	
Picornavirus family	Poliovirus
Enterovirus genus	Coxsackievirus Echovirus Enteroviruses 70 and 71
Parechovirus genus	Parechoviruses 1 and 2 (formerly echoviruses 22 and 23)
Hepatovirus genus	Hepatitis A virus
Togavirus family	
Alphavirus genus (arbovirus)	Equine encephalitis (eastern, western, Venezuela)
Rubivirus genus	Rubella virus
Flavivirus family and genus (arbovirus)	St Louis encephalitis Japanese encephalitis Tick-borne encephalitis West Nile virus
Bunyavirus family (arbovirus)	California encephalitis
Reovirus family (arbovirus)	Colorado tick fever (coltivirus)
Orthomyxovirus family	Influenza A and B viruses
Paramyxovirus family	Measles and subacute sclerosing panencephalitis Mumps
Arenavirus family and genus	Lymphocytic choriomeningitis
Rhabdovirus family	Rabies
Retrovirus family	HIV, AIDS Human T-cell lymphotropic virus (HAM/TSP)
DNA viruses	
Herpesvirus family	HSV Varicella zoster (virus) CMV EBV, infectious mononucleosis Human herpesvirus 6–8
Papovavirus family	Progressive multifocal leukoencephalopathy
Poxvirus family	Vaccinia virus
Adenovirus family	Adenovirus

Abbreviations: CMV, cytomegalovirus; EBV, Epstein-Barr virus; HAM, human T-cell lymphotropic virus type 1–associated myelopathy; HIV, human immunodeficiency virus; HSV, herpes simplex virus; TSP, tropical spastic paraparesis.
From Rowland LP, Pedley TA. Merritt's neurology. Philadelphia: Wolters Kluwer; 2009. p. 157; with permission.

diagnosis.[1] Although it is usually caused by certain viruses it also has several other origins, both infectious and noninfectious, and the advent of polymerase chain reaction (PCR) testing has greatly improved the determination of specific causes in most cases of aseptic meningitis.[2]

Epidemiology

There are multiple organisms that cause viral meningitis. No specific pattern appears to be associated with this disorder, although seasonal aspects do play a significant part in its spread. Enteroviruses encompass approximately more than 70 serotypes, which cause more than 85% of all cases of viral meningitis.[2] These viruses are spread from person to person by the fecal-oral and respiratory routes, and are found in the summer and late fall in moderate climates. The adenovirus is spread via the respiratory route and from reactivation of a latent virus, causing meningitis in immunocompromised individuals. Lymphocytic choriomeningitis is transmitted to humans from direct contact with rodents. Varicella (chickenpox) is latent many years after exposure to the virus. Herpes can be spread from person to person via epithelial contact or sexual contact.

Etiology

The principal viruses identified with meningitis are enteroviruses (Coxsackievirus, echovirus, and poliovirus), herpes simplex types 1 (HSV-1) and 2 (HSV-2), varicella zoster virus (VZV), paramyxoviruses (mumps), arenaviruses (lymphocytic choriomeningitis), and adenovirus. Most viral infections of the CNS are uncommon complications of a systemic illnesses caused by common human pathogens. After multiplication of the virus in the extraneural tissues, the virus disseminates to the CNS by the hematologic route or is spread along the nerve fibers.[3]

Clinical Manifestations

The determination of the causative agent depends on a review of the epidemiologic features, clinical assessment, and laboratory findings. The onset of illness is generally acute, although it can be insidious over the course of a week.[2] Fever (<102.0 F/39 C), headache, nuchal rigidity, and altered mental status are key symptoms of meningitis. However, the clinical presence of these symptoms should not allow the health care provider to solely rely on the clinical characteristics alone, diagnostic evaluation being imperative.[4] Brudzinski and Kerning signs may be apparent. Muscle weakness is rarely reported, but myalgia is present.

Diagnosis

Accurate diagnosis relies on the clinical picture and epidemiology of the individual. The classic symptomatology of meningitis leads practitioners to perform a lumbar puncture to identify bacteria or viruses and the differential count of leukocytes. The diagnosis of an acute viral infection and establishment of the type of virus rests on the development of antibodies to the infection, traditionally a 4-fold antibody increase. It is therefore necessary to show that antibodies are not present or are present in low titer in the first few days of the illness, and are present in high titer 3 to 5 weeks after the onset of illness. When there is no change in titer, positive tests merely indicate that the individual at some time in the past had an infection with this type of virus and that it is probably not the cause of the present illness.[3]

Cerebrospinal fluid (CSF) specimens should transported to the laboratory and processed promptly to avoid depletion of cell counts that may hinder an accurate diagnosis. In viral meningitis, the cell count does not exceed 1000 white blood cells per cubic millimeter.[1] The classic finding in viral meningitis is predominance of small lymphocytes, and polymorphonuclear (PMN) leukocytes may predominate for the first 24 to 48 hours. Protein counts are normal but may be elevated, and glucose is usually normal. Of the many viruses that can cause meningitis, only some enteroviruses can be cultured readily from CSF.[1] Adding to the diagnostics is the utilization of PCR assays, which add a high degree of sensitivity and a quicker diagnosis for the physician. Lactic acid is usually normal. Elevated levels of lactic acid coupled with other CSF findings can be found in partially treated meningitis.

Most risk factors for meningitis can be guided by the "6 I's"[4]:

1. Infection (urinary tract or lower infection, sinusitis, otitis)
2. Immunosuppression (splenectomy, sickle cell, human immunodeficiency virus [HIV])
3. Injury (head trauma, neurologic or otolaryngologic procedures)
4. Indwelling catheters
5. Imbiber
6. Identification

Important data for encephalitis can be obtained through the use of the "6 V's"[4]:

1. Vacation/travel: to endemic areas, foreign or domestic
2. Veterinary or other animal contact
3. Vectors: recent mosquito or tick bites
4. Viral infections: recent or concurrent
5. Vaccinations: recent for measles, rubella, varicella, or rabies
6. Vital statistics: contact local agencies for outbreaks

Viral meningitis itself is not associated with findings on imaging.[5] Magnetic resonance imaging (MRI) findings may only show inflammation of the brain and/or spinal cord.

Causes

Enteroviruses

Enteroviruses are found in mucus, saliva, and feces, and are transmitted through direct contact with infected persons, objects, or surfaces. Because they are heat-resistant and acid-resistant, transmission is increased in the hotter months. Enteroviruses are the most common cause of aseptic meningitis.[6] Headache, usually frontal to orbital, is seen along with photophobia, fever, and meningeal signs. CSF leukocytes are mildly increased. The duration of the illness lasts from 1 to 2 weeks.

Coxsackievirus

The coxsackievirus was discovered by accident in 1948 in a suspected polio patient and was named after the town in New York where it was isolated. This group includes poliovirus, echovirus, and coxsackievirus A and B, infections and most recently viruses that are designated by number, such as enterovirus 71.[5] Organism identification is key to the connection and surveillance of outbreaks when they occur.

Group A coxsackievirus is distinguished in the manner whereby it manifests in newborn mice. Extraneural signs and symptoms are herpangina, hand-foot-mouth disease, and rashes. Group B coxsackievirus causes pericarditis, myocarditis, and epidemic myalgia.[3] In early pregnancy, exposed infants may have disseminated infection and various congenital anomalies. However, in humans both groups can cause aseptic meningitis and, rarely, encephalitis.

Signs and symptoms are similar, with fever, headache, malaise, nausea, and abdominal pain. Stiff neck and vomiting occur after 24 to 48 hours. CSF pressures are normal to slightly increased, with moderate pleocytosis from PMN cells initially. Within 12 to 24 hours a switch to primary lymphocytes is seen. Protein is normal to slightly increased, with a normal glucose count.

Diagnosis is established by virus identification from feces, throat washings, CSF, or antibodies in serum. Treatment is supportive, and for prevention or containment of outbreaks thorough hand washing and personal protective equipment (PPE) are used.

Echoviruses

Echoviruses were first isolated from apparently normal individuals. The organisms were considered "orphans" in that they were not thought to cause disease. Echo is an acronym for Enteric Crypto pathogenic Human Orphans (ECHO). This virus causes gastroenteritis, macular exanthemas, and upper respiratory infections. Echovirus-9 causes a petichial rash that is often confused with meningococcemia. When the CNS is involved, aseptic meningitis develops.[3]

Children are more affected than adults, the main symptoms being fever, sore throat, vomiting, and diarrhea. When the nervous system is involved, headache, neck stiffness, irritability, and lethargy are present. It runs a course of 1 to 2 weeks with complications similar to those of coxsackievirus. If a persistent CNS infection is present, agammaglobulinemia can result.

Diagnosis is from CSF pleocytosis, varying from several hundred to thousand or more cells per cubic millimeter. Early infections may show 90% PMN leukocytes. Viral typing is done by antibody testing with additional genomic amplification.[3] Treatment is supportive, with thorough hand washing and PPE used as for coxsackievirus outbreaks.

Poliovirus

Poliovirus infections present with a more myelitic pattern, affecting the spinal cord and brainstem. The symptomatology is flaccid muscle paralysis of muscles throughout the body as it affects the large motor cells; degeneration of the neurons leads to an inflammatory response, and recovery occurs in partially damaged cells. Of the 3 defined types of poliovirus, type 1 is most associated with paralytic disease. The inactivated poliovirus vaccine is the one used most often, because the oral vaccine contains a live attenuated virus capable of vaccine-associated poliomyelitis. The symptoms start with fever, chills, and nausea. The symptoms subside in 36 to 48 hours, then an increase in temperature is seen with symptoms of meningeal irritation. Paralysis is noted around the second to fifth day, affecting the limbs and the respiratory muscles. Diagnostic data show an increase in leukocytosis in the blood. A lumbar puncture is performed with increased pressures present. Pleocytosis is noted in the period before paralysis is noted. CSF protein is elevated except in those with severe paralysis, and stays elevated for weeks.

The diagnosis is rendered because of the acute development of asymmetric flaccid paralysis with the changes in CSF, along with a history if nonvaccination or presentation with a weak immune response. The virus can be recovered in stool specimens (lasting 2–3 weeks) and throat washings during the first week. A 4-fold increase in the antibody titer is required in the stool and throat washings before a specific diagnosis can be made. PCR is found to be positive. Poliovirus is rarely found is CSF and blood specimens.

Treatment is supportive for the patient, with care given to the respiratory, swallowing, bowel, and bladder functions. The virus has an affinity to the late summer and early fall. Before the discovery of the poliomyelitis vaccine in 1965, it was the most common form of viral infection.[3]

Herpes

Both HSV-1 and HSV-2 can cause CNS infections. HSV-1 is more likely to cause aseptic meningitis. Herpes virus of the CNS can be a result of a primary or recurrent reinfection, although it is implicated more as a complication of a primary infection.[1] HSV meningitis accounts for approximately 10% of acute viral meningitis in adults.[7] The absence of a herpetic lesion does not exclude the possibility of CNS involvement of HSV. Herpes meningitis has a better prognosis than encephalitis and is almost self-limiting, without lasting issues. HSV now ranks as the second most common cause of viral meningitis in adolescents and adults in developed countries.[8] HSV-2 meningitis may be present in the absence of clinical genital herpes.[5]

HSV-2 meningitis can recur in women with primary genital infection. HSV-2 and herpes simplex type antibodies have been detected in CSF of 85% of patients.[9] Type 2 infection in the adult more typically causes an aseptic meningitis and sometimes polyradiculitis or myelitis, usually with a recent genital herpes infection. There are multiple diagnoses that can mimic HSV meningitis, and early recognition is imperative. Rapid use of acyclovir has been shown to be an effective therapy. HSV was previously diagnosed via brain biopsy, but PCR testing is now the definitive means of diagnosis.

Mollaret meningitis is a rare form of meningitis that is recurrent, aseptic, and self-limiting, and should be considered in all persons with recurrent aseptic meningitis. HSV-2 has been thought to be a recurring organism in this type of meningitis.[10] The course of the disease, although prolonged, is benign, and does not pose a threat to the patient. Early diagnosis can prevent repeated hospitalizations and exhaustive workups. In general, the symptoms tend to recur over a period of 3 to 5 years, although a case lasting longer than 28 years has been reported.[11] Acyclovir administered intravenously or orally, or valacyclovir given orally is the treatment of choice.

Varicella zoster virus

Approximately 95% of the adult population has been infected with VZV following an initial infection with varicella (chickenpox). The primary VZV infection presents in an immunocompromised patient, causing meningitis or encephalitis.[7] Typical presentation is with acute focal deficits and ataxia, owing to the large vascular distribution that follows the trigeminal nerve. Rash may not be present. Multifocal ischemic and hemorrhagic infarcts are seen on imaging, and diagnosis is finalized by PCR assay. CSF findings are is indistinguishable from those of other viral meningitides. Therapy is supportive, and acyclovir and steroids have been shown to help.

Mumps

This disorder is caused by the paramyxovirus, which has an affinity for the salivary glands, pancreas, breast, mature gonads, and the nervous system.[3] It is spread via droplets from the respiratory system. CNS involvement occurring with a mild form of meningitis or encephalitis is uncommon. With mumps meningitis, the virus is known to replicate in the choroidal and ependymal cells, whereas in encephalitis it results from direct action of the virus or from an immune-mediated demyelination. Mumps has a low mortality rate, thus its pathology is unclear. Before the vaccine era, the most common form of meningoencephalitis, accounting for approximately 10% of cases.[1] With the advent of the mumps vaccine, the number of infections was drastically reduced. The infection should be considered in males who develop an aseptic meningitis in the winter or spring months.

Mumps CNS syndromes are more common in older groups and should be suspected in males, who are affected 3 times more often and who develop aseptic meningitis in the winter or spring months.[12] A definitive history of mumps aids the practitioner in excluding the disease, as a previous attack confers lifelong immunity.[12]

Deafness, mainly unilateral, is the most common side effect of mumps. Other symptoms such as myelitis, optic neuritis, and other cranial nerve (CN) palsies may present 7 to 15 days after onset.

Lymphocytic choriomeningitis

This virus was first described by Wallgren in 1925 as aseptic meningitis. It was the first whereby a virus was proved to be the cause of a benign meningitis with a predominance of lymphocytes in the CSF.[3] It causes less than 0.5% of cases of viral meningitis.[1] Human-to-human transmission has only occurred through maternal-fetal transmission and solid organ transplantation. Microencephaly, mental retardation epilepsy, and cerebral palsy are common long-lasting effects. Rodents and mice are colonized with this virus, which is excreted in urine and feces. Its peak may occur at any time with the exception of the summer months. Key to the health care professional is possible exposure of the patient to rodents.

Onset of infection is characterized by fever, headache, malaise, myalgia, and symptoms of upper respiratory infection. Meningeal symptoms may occur 1 week after onset. Severe headache, nausea, and vomiting mark the beginning of neurologic involvement. Definitive diagnosis may be made by recovery of the virus from blood or CSF, mainly by serology and immunoglobulin M (IgM) antibodies. Duration of symptoms lasts 1 to 4 weeks; mortality is low and fatality less than 1%. Complete recovery is seen, though rarely in those with encephalitis with residual focal lesions in brain and spinal cord. No definitive treatment has been recognized.

Adenovirus

This virus was not discovered until 1953 when it was isolated from tissue culture from surgically removed tonsils and adenoids, hence the name. Adenovirus is found in patients who may be immunocompromised as a result of kidney or bone marrow transplantation It commonly takes the form of meningoencephalitis. It is spread by the respiratory and gastrointestinal routes and causes a variety of syndromes. Most infections occur in children, with 50% being asymptomatic. Neurologic involvement is found in children. Only a few pathologic studies have been done, and the encephalitis appears to be of the primary type with viral invasion of the brain. The encephalitis is moderate to severe with lethargy, ataxia confusion, coma, and death. CSF pleocytosis is evident, and PMN or mononuclear leukocytes are present. Diagnosis made by serology or by isolation of virus from CSF, throat, respiratory tract, and feces. No specific treatment has been determined.

ENCEPHALITIS

Distinguishing meningitis syndromes from encephalitis can be difficult. Encephalitis presents with seizures, altered level of consciousness, and focal neurologic deficits involving the brain parenchyma only. There are 2 types of encephalitis: primary encephalitis (acute viral encephalitis), caused by direct viral infection of the brain, and spinal cord and secondary encephalitis (postinfective encephalitis), which results from complications of a current viral infection.

Epidemiology

Epidemiologically there are two distinct patterns. The first is identical to meningitis in that it involves respiratory or oral person-to-person transmission. The other is typical of an arboviral diseases, requires direct injection of the virus into the bloodstream through a bite of an infected insect, such as a mosquito or tick.[1] Intermediate hosts have been identified as horses or birds. Humans are identified as incidental or "dead-end" hosts. Epidemiologic clues can assist the physician in directing care for the eventual diagnosis; these may include season of the year, geographic location, local prevalence within the community, travel history, recreational activities, insect/animal contact, vaccine history, and the immune status of the patient.[13] **Table 2**

Table 2
Epidemiologic characteristics and laboratory diagnosis of viral encephalitis

Virus	Recent Travel	Risky Habitat	Month of Exposure	Patient Age	Diagnostic Test	Research Laboratory
St Louis encephalitis	United States	Unscreened home	Jun–Aug	Older	IgM ELISA	CDC
Japanese encephalitis	Asia	Rice fields	May–Sep	Any	IgM ELISA	WRAIR
Eastern equine encephalitis	Western North America, South America	Agroecosystems in western United States	Jun–Sep	Any	IgM ELISA	CDC
Eastern equine encephalitis	Eastern United States	Coastal marshland	Jun–Aug	<10, >55 y	IgM ELISA	CDC
Venezuelan equine encephalitis	South America to Texas	Rural	Rainy months	Adult men	IgM ELISA CSF	CDC
Tick-borne encephalitis	Central Europe and Asia	Woodlands	Jun–Aug	Any	IgM ELISA CSF	U. Vienna
Herpes simplex	Anywhere	None	Any	Any	Brain biopsy	
California encephalitis	Western United States	Rural areas	Jun–Oct	Children	IgM ELISA	CDC
Murray Valley encephalitis	Southern Australia	River valley area	Jan–May	Any	IgM ELISA	CDC
West Nile encephalitis	North Africa, eastern and southern Asia East coast of United States	Rice areas New York City metropolitan area	Jun–Sep Jun–Sep	Any Any	ELISA virus isolation PCR, virus isolation	WRAIR Most
Powassan	North central United States, southern Canada	Rural areas	Jun–Sep	<20 or >50 y	HAI, CF	CDC
La Crosse	Midwestern United States	Woodlands	Jun–Sep	Boys <19 y	ELISA	CDC
Rocio	Sao Paulo, Brazil	Poor rural areas	Feb–Jul	Young men	HAI, ELISA	CDC
Jamestown Canyon	New York and Westward	Rural areas	Jun–Sep	Children	CF, NT	
HIV type 1	Worldwide	All	Any	Undefined	ELISA immunoblot	Most
B virus		Monkey colony	Any	Adult	Virus isolation	SFBR

Abbreviations: CDC laboratory, Fort Collins, CO; CF, complement fixation; CSF, cerebrospinal fluid; ELISA, enzyme-linked immunosorbent assay; HAI, hemagglutination inhibition; IgM, immunoglobulin M; NT, neutralization test; PCR, polymerase chain reaction; SFBR, Southwest Foundation for Biomedical Research, San Antonio, TX; U. Vienna, University of Vienna, Vienna, Austria; WRAIR, Department of Viral Diseases, Walter Reed Army Institute of Research, Washington, DC.
From Gorbach SL, Bartlett JG, Blacklow NR. Infectious diseases. Philadelphia: Wolters Kluwer; 2003. p. 1290; with permission.

demonstrates the various epidemiologic characteristics of the various viruses and demonstrates the variety of season, geographic location, and climatic conditions.

Etiology

The viruses causing encephalitis have an arboviral pattern of origin or are caused by the bite of a vector such as an insect or infected mammal. **Table 3** summarizes the modes of transmission for specific encephalitis syndromes.

Clinical Manifestations

Periods of incubation are difficult to calculate precisely in the case of animal bites. In arboviral cases, incubation can vary from several days to 2 weeks. Although most arboviral infections (>90%) result in an influenza-type illness, with encephalitis the syndrome generally consists of fever, headache, malaise, and altered mental status. Nuchal rigidity and seizures may occur. Within the first week paralysis may be flaccid or spastic, and many patients exhibit symptoms of syndrome of inappropriate antidiuretic hormone (SIADH). The patient will progress, and will either show signs of improvement or expire. The lasting side effects of the disease are CN and cognitive deficits, if present.

Diagnosis

A complete evaluation includes complete blood count, hepatic and renal function tests, coagulation studies, and chest radiography. Neuroimaging can document intracranial abnormality.[13] CSF analysis is essential (unless contraindicated) for an encephalitis workup, and will show mild to moderate pleocytosis. Protein levels may be slightly elevated, with glucose being essentially normal. Erythrocytes found in CSF may be common in HSV encephalitis, owing to hemorrhagic lesions in the parenchyma of the brain.

Table 3
Grouping and mode of transmission of encephalitis viruses

Family	Member Virus	Transmission (Vector)
Flaviviridae	Japanese encephalitis	
	St Louis encephalitis	
	Murray Valley encephalitis	*Culex* mosquitos
	West Nile encephalitis	
	Powassan	*Ixodes* ticks
	Tick-borne encephalitis	
Togaviridae (alphaviruses)	Eastern equine encephalitis	
	Western equine encephalitis	
	Venezuelan equine encephalitis	*Culex* mosquitos
Bunyaviridae	California group	
	La Crosse	*Aedes* mosquitos
	Jamestown Canyon	
Herpesviridae	HSV-1 > HSV-2	Person to person
	Cytomegalovirus	Person to person
	Varicella-zoster	Person to person
	Monkey B	Monkey bite
Retroviridae	HIV type 1	Person to person

From Gorbach SL, Bartlett JG, Blacklow NR. Infectious diseases. Philadelphia: Wolters Kluwer; 2003. p. 1290; with permission.

A check for IgM antibodies can identify specific agents. Rapid detection and identification can be accomplished with PCR because of its accuracy, especially for herpes and enteroviruses.[13] Ancillary tests may help to confirm, but not establish, a cause. Electroencephalography (EEG) is most sensitive early in infection and may show slow focal waves over the affected brain. Computed tomography (CT) of the brain is insensitive early in infection, and MRI is more sensitive to soft-tissue abnormalities.

Treatment

Acyclovir should be initiated in all patients suspected with encephalitis, pending diagnostic results.[13] The only form of viral encephalitis for which there is effective treatment available is caused by the herpesvirus.[1] Once the cause of encephalitis has been identified, specific antimicrobial therapy should be used for that infectious agent or therapy should be discontinued if an agent is not found. At present, supportive care in encephalitis patients for nutrition, venous thromboembolism (VTE), respiratory infections and therapies assist patients in obtaining a functional status. **Fig. 1** shows an evaluation and treatment algorithm.

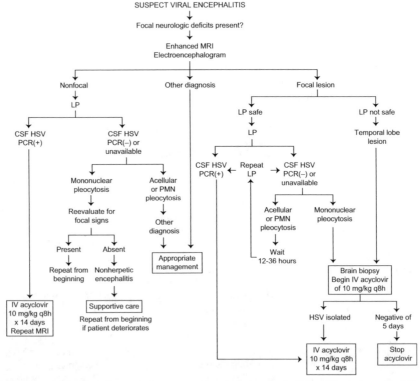

Fig. 1. Algorithm to evaluate and treat suspected viral encephalitis. CSF, cerebrospinal fluid; HSV, herpes simplex virus; IV, intravenous; LP, lumbar puncture; MRI, magnetic resonance imaging; PCR, polymerase chain reaction; PMN, polymorphonuclear leukocytes. (*From* Johnson RT, Griffin JW. Current therapy in neurologic disease. 5th edition. St Louis (MO): Mosby; 1997. p. 158; with permission.)

Prevention

Because there is no effective therapy for most causes of viral encephalitis, vaccines are desirable. Vaccines have been developed for Japanese B, Venezuelan, and tick-borne encephalitides, but only the Japanese B is available in the United States. The best course is measures to prevent exposure to mosquito or tick vectors. Mumps and measles vaccines have markedly decreased the incidence of encephalitis. Rabies vaccine is effective in preventing disease even after the bite of an infected animal.[1]

Causes

Herpes simplex virus

HSV encephalitis is the most commonly diagnosed encephalitis in industrialized nations. Herpes is a DNA-containing virus, and the members of this group establish latent infections over a long period. It arises sporadically or only when a trigger reactivates an infection.[3] HSV encephalitis is rarely seen as an opportunistic infection. Diagnosis has been greatly improved with CSF PCR, and has expanded the awareness of mild or atypical encephalitis.

HSV-1 is transmitted by respiratory or salivary contact. The primary infection occurs in childhood or adolescence. It usually presents subclinically, and approximately 50% of the population have an antibody to HSV-1 by the age of 15 years, whereas 50% to 90% of adults have the antibody depending on socioeconomic status.[3] It occurs mainly in adults older than 20 years and occurs from endogenous reactivation of the virus in relation to a primary exposure.[3] In reactivation, neurologic involvement is rare. However, during primary infection the virus becomes latent in the trigeminal ganglia. At a later time a stimulus can reactivate the virus, which is usually seen as herpes labialis (cold sores). The virus reaches the brain through the branches of the trigeminal nerve to the basal meninges, resulting in a localization of encephalitis to the temporal and orbital frontal lobes.

HSV-2 is spread through sexual contact except in the case of infantile infection during delivery.[3] It can cause aseptic meningitis in adults, is often the primary infection, and can occur with reactivation.

Symptoms that evolve over days are headache, fever, seizures, confusion, stupor, and coma. Onset is most often abrupt, and may be seen with focal or major motor seizures. The encephalitis evolves much more slowly, with aphasia and mental changes preceding more ominous neurologic symptoms. Some patients have stated that the manifestations are preceded by symptoms that include gustatory and olfactory hallucinations. Other symptoms are anosmia, temporal lobe seizures, personality changes, bizarre behavior, delirium, aphasia, and hemiparesis.[12] Status epilepticus is a rare finding. A history of cold sores is not helpful in making the diagnosis because the incidence is similar to that of the general population.[3]

CSF shows mild pressure and pleocytosis. Lymphocytic cells are found as well as a significant number of neutrophils. Protein count is elevated, with glucose rarely less than 40 mg/dL. The lesions take form as hemorrhagic necrosis of the inferior border medial temporal lobes and medio-orbital parts of the frontal lobes. Temporal lesions are bilateral but not symmetric. The localization of these lesions in HSV encephalitis has been supposedly explained by the virus' route of entry into the CNS.[12] Two routes have been suggested. The virus is thought to be latent in the trigeminal ganglia and to infect the nose and the olfactory tract on reactivation. Alternatively, with reactivation the trigeminal neuralgia the infection may spread along the nerve fibers that innervate the leptomeninges of the anterior and posterior fossa. The lack of lesions in the olfactory bulbs in as many as 40% of fatal cases is a point in favor of the second pathway.[12]

CT shows hypodensity of the affected areas in 50% to 60% of cases but cannot be relied on in early diagnosis, and MRI shows signal changes in almost all images. It has become general practice to initiate acyclovir until confirmatory testing is completed. Acyclovir is dosed at 30 mg/kg/d and is continued for 10 to 14 days to prevent relapse. Definitive diagnosis may be established by recovery of the virus from the CSF (rare) or brain, PCR, or viral antigens in the brain.[3]

The outcome of the disease depends to a large extent on the patient's age and state of consciousness at the time acyclovir is initiated. Herpes responds well before coma develops, and early with the administration of acyclovir. Without treatment the disease is fatal in 70% to 80% of cases, and those who survive the acute disease are left with severe neurologic residuals. Survival is greater than 90% if treatment is started within 4 days of the onset of illness.[12]

Arboviruses

These small, spherical RNA-enveloped viruses are spread most commonly via a blood-sucking vector such as a mosquito or tick. Birds are the principal hosts, but humans and horses are usually incidental hosts and are also dead-end hosts. Outbreaks occur in hotter months and when crowded conditions or large populations of infected vectors are present.[3]

Arboviral encephalitis has a global distribution.[14] There are 4 common causes of mosquito-transmitted encephalitis in the United States: (1) Equine (eastern equine encephalitis [EEE], western equine encephalitis [WEE], and Venezuelan equine encephalitis [VEE]); (2) La Crosse encephalitis; (3) St Louis encephalitis (SLE); and (4) West Nile virus (WNV). Most of such viruses are asymptomatic or present with a nonspecific influenza-like syndrome.

Prevention can occur through decreasing time outdoors during early evening hours, wearing long pants and shirts, and applying mosquito repellent to areas of exposed skin. The spraying of insecticide in areas where mosquitoes lay their eggs is often carried out to kill juvenile larvae and adult mosquitoes.

Surveillance is becoming increasingly refined to allow for rapid detection and identification, thus to decrease the threat to public health, shorten public health response time, and reduce the geographic spread and cost of containing the virus.[14] The Arbovirus Diseases Branch of the National Center for Infectious Diseases Division of Vector Borne Infectious Diseases has the responsibility for the Centers for Disease Control and Prevention (CDC) programs in surveillance, diagnosis, research, and control of arboviral encephalitides.[14]

The virus is difficult to locate in the laboratory and can be recovered in blood during the early phase (2–4 days) of illness.

Equine encephalitis

Eastern equine encephalitis It is imperative to distinguish equine encephalitis from other acute CNS infections. EEE was identified in the 1930s and occurs in focal areas of the Eastern seaboard, the Gulf Coast, and some areas of the Midwest. The EEE virus occurs in natural cycles in birds in swampy areas during warm months. It is unknown as to where the virus resides or its survival in the winter. It is thought to be introduced by migratory birds in spring, and can remain dormant in some as yet unknown parts of the life cycle. It remains unknown as to why the virus escapes the focus of the birds in swampy areas and moves to other vectors such as *Coquilletidia perturbans* and *Aedes sollicitans*, which do feed on mammals and birds that ultimately transmit the virus to humans and horses. Equine vaccines are available. When local health officials maintain surveillance for the movement out of the swampy areas, and the level is sufficiently increased, measures are taken to reduce the risk to humans.[15] Ten cases were reported in 2010 in the United States.[16]

EEE is a rare infection of humans, and tends to occur in small epidemics or small outbreaks. Human cases of EEE are usually preceded by cases in horses, which is used as a surveillance tool. EEE mainly affects children, infants, and adults older than 50 years.

Symptoms begin with short duration (5 days) of fever, headache, malaise, and nausea/vomiting that occur 4 to 10 days after the bite from an infected mosquito. There is a rapid neurologic onset of manifestations: confusion, drowsiness, stupor, or convulsive seizures. CN palsies and hemiplegia are common.

In EEE the brain is markedly congested on autopsy, with widespread degenerative changes in nerve cells. There are massive destructive lesions involving a major part of a lobe or hemisphere, seen easily on MRI, whereas in other arboviruses the foci are relatively small.

Leukocytosis in particular will be noted in blood in EEE. CSF changes are greatest in EEE, with pressure moderately or greatly increased. CSF is cloudy or purulent with 500 to 3000 cells per cubic centimeter; PMN leukocytes are also predominant. The isolation of equine encephalitis from blood and CSF is infrequent. Most arboviral infections are diagnosed serologically, with IgM assays available for rapid diagnosis.

Mortality averages about 50% in EEE. Recovered patients have mental deficiency, CN palsies, hemiplegia, aphasia, and convulsions. Children younger than 10 years are more likely to survive the infection, but also have the greatest chance of lifelong neurosequelae.

Treatment is supportive in the acute phase. Vaccines have been produced but are confined for use usually to laboratory workers and others who have a high level of exposure to the virus. Because of the low incidence, large-scale vaccination is not warranted for the public.

Western equine encephalitis WEE is another alphavirus discovered in the 1930s, and was first isolated from the brain of a horse with encephalitis.[14] The infection is apparent in the birds and *Culex tarsalis* associated with irrigated agriculture and stream drainage.[17,18]

Human cases are usually found in June or July and the infection is asymptomatic or presents as a mild, nonspecific illness. WEE is less intense, and is characterized by less inflammation and a paucity of nerve cell changes.[3] Fulminant illness is seen with sudden-onset fever, headache, nausea/vomiting, anorexia, and malaise, followed by altered level of consciousness and signs of meningeal irritation. Children younger than 1 year are most affected, more severely than adults, and 5% to 30% of patients are left with permanent sequelae. Mortality is 3%.

Venezuelan equine encephalitis VEE causes encephalitis to horses and humans, and is a public health and veterinary issue in Central and South America. The natural reservoir host for the strain is not known. The virus is maintained in forests with cycles involving forest-dwelling rodents and mosquito vectors, mainly *Culex (Melanoconion)* species. The most recent epidemic of VEE occurred in 1995 in Venezuela and Columbia, with an estimated 90,000 infections.[14] The infection of humans is less severe in VEE than in EEE or WEE, and fatalities are rare. Adults present with an influenza-type illness and children usually develop encephalitis. There are effective equine vaccines available.

La Crosse encephalitis La Crosse encephalitis was discovered in La Crosse, Wisconsin, in 1963.[14] In 2010 80 cases were reported in the United States, with the majority being children.[19] Is found in the eastern half of the continental United States. Transmitted by the woodland *Aedes triseriatus* mosquito, the cycle involves small woodland animals such as chipmunks and squirrels as intermediate hosts. La Crosse occurs in late summer and fall, and usually affects infants. Incubation is 5 to 15 days. Symptoms are headache, nausea/vomiting, changes in sensorium, seizures, and meningeal irritation. Encephalitis is usually mild. Diagnosis is by increased number of lymphocytes in CSF, as well as serologic tests and genomic amplification.[3] Fatality is low (<1%) and recovery takes place within 7 to 10 days. Emotional ability, learning difficulties, and recurrent seizures have been reported after recovery. In clinical settings, pediatric cases are routinely screened for herpes or enteroviral etiology. There is no specific treatment. Most physicians do not specifically request identification of the La Crosse virus, and most cases are reported as aseptic meningitis or viral encephalitis of unknown etiology.[14]

St Louis Encephalitis The first outbreak of this encephalitis was in 1933, in St Louis, Missouri. The virus is a mosquito-transmitted flavivirus and follows 2 patterns: rural and urban. No cases were reported in 2010 in the United States.[20]

SLE is the most common mosquito-transmitted human pathogen in the United States.[14] It is distributed throughout the lower 48 states, although periodic outbreaks have occurred in the Midwest and Southeast. Less than 1% of the outbreaks of SLE or clinically apparent, and the vast majority go undiagnosed. The illness can range from simple febrile headache to meningoencephalitis, with an overall fatality of 5% to 15%. It is milder in children than in adults, but those children who do have the virus have a higher rate of encephalitis.[14] The elderly are at highest risk of severe disease and death. During the summer, the virus is maintained in a mosquito-bird-mosquito cycle, with periods of amplification in domestic birds and *Culex* mosquitoes.[14] The mosquito species varies from region to region in the United States. Urban outbreaks are abrupt and extensive, as the virus tends to replicate in urban mosquitoes. About 75% of patients with clinical manifestations have encephalitis, and others have aseptic meningitis or aspecific illness. Onset of symptoms may be abrupt or preceded by prodromal illness of 3 to 4 days' duration, characterized by headache that increases with severity, fever, myalgias, sore throat, and nausea/vomiting. Other common symptoms are ataxia, CN abnormalities, confusion, and intention tremor. With more severe cases, delirium, coma, stupor, and seizures result, which are considered poor prognostic signs.

CSF has mild leukocytosis with lymphocytes being the predominant cell type, and PMN cells may be found early in the disease. Glucose is normal and hyponatremia arises from SIADH in 25% to 33% of patients.[3] SLE is rarely isolated in blood or CSF, and diagnosis depends on serologic testing. The areas of the thalamus and midbrain are more affected than the cerebral cortex.

The disease runs an acute course, and either death or recovery occurs within 2 to 3 weeks. Mortality is between 2% and 20%.[3] For several years after diagnosis, patients have reported sequelae such as headache, insomnia, irritability, and memory loss, which eventually clears. About 25% of survivors have permanent neurologic issues such as CN palsies, gait disorders, and aphasia. Supportive care is essential, as there is no specific treatment available. Preventive treatment is through vector control and avoidance of the vectors that spread the disease.

West Nile virus This flavivirus is related to SLE and Japanese encephalitis, and is endemic to Africa, the Middle East, and Southwest Asia. It is not known by which mechanism WNV spread to North America. It was first recognized in the late summer of 1999 when there was an outbreak in New York City. The only known vector is the

Culex mosquito. The rapidity of the virus' spread led to the suggestion that it was facilitated by migratory birds. However, newer modes of transmission have been identified in transmission via breast milk from the nursing mother to the newborn, transplanted organs and blood products from infected donors, and placenta from pregnant mother to fetus.[1]

According to the CDC as of November 27, 2012, 48 states have reported approximately 5204 cases of WNV, with 234 deaths. Of these 5204 cases, 51% were neuroinvasive cases and 49% were not neuroinvasive. Eighty percent of the cases were reported in the states of Texas (which has a reported one-third of cases), California, Louisiana, Illinois, Michigan, South Dakota, Oklahoma, Nebraska, Colorado, Arizona, Ohio, and New York.[21]

Most WNV infections remain asymptomatic. Approximately 20% of infected individuals develop an acute influenza-like illness, and only 1 in 150 develop neuroinvasive disease. Patients tend to be older than 60 years, and immunosuppression, hypertension, diabetes, and liver disease are comorbidities linked to the development of a neuroinvasive nature and poor prognosis.

A special syndrome of febrile, flaccid paralytic poliomyelitis resulting from WNV is now well known, which evolves over several days and in a few cases has led to extrapyramidal syndromes.

The pathologic changes in WNV are consistent with widespread degeneration of the single nerve cells as well as scattered foci of inflammatory necrosis.[12] The brainstem is relatively spared. WNV has a regional pattern of damage, and usually affects the anterior horns of the spinal cord as well leading to poliomyelitis, as previously stated.

WNV is clinically similar to other forms of aseptic meningitis, and is characterized by headache, nuchal rigidity, and photophobia. In approximately 20% of cases CN palsies, particularly of the facial nerve, occur. CSF shows pleocytosis, elevated protein, and normal glucose level. Imaging studies are normal. With encephalitis the patient will experience headache, changes in mental status, and movement disorders with myoclonus, tremor, parkinsonism, ataxia, and weakness. CSF findings are similar to those of meningitis.

Diagnosis for WNV is based on serologic testing. After infection the patient may have serum immunoglobulin G antibodies for life, indicating past exposure. In the acute phase, IgM are found and are still present 3 months after infection in almost all patients, and in 60% to 70% of patients 18 months after infection; 20% of cases still have detectable serum IgM antibodies 18 months after infection.[22] Detection of CSF WNV IgM antibodies is diagnostic of neuroinvasive WNV disease. The large size of the IgM molecules means they cross the blood-brain barrier poorly and, as a result, findings in the CSF generally indicate intrathecal synthesis.[22] Reverse transcriptase PCR of CSF is highly specific but relatively insensitive in the diagnosis of neuroinvasive disease. CT of the brain may show normal findings.

There has been no proven beneficial treatment for WNV, although supportive care remains beneficial. The infection has an acute course over 2 to 3 weeks. Dementia and paralysis are the most frequent residuals. Vector control, repellent, and protective clothing are preventive measures.

Rabies

Rabies is often underreported, so it is difficult to obtain an accurate number of cases worldwide. It is found mainly in underdeveloped countries.[23] There were two confirmed cases of rabies in the United States in 2010, one in Louisiana from a patient who acquired the disease from a rabid bat in Mexico before immigrating to the United States for work. The other case, in Wisconsin, was attributed to a domestic acquisition from a bat as well.[24] A rabies variant had been found in a US soldier returning from war who eventually died 3 months after exposure. Thus according to the CDC (2012), post-deployment evaluations by the Department of Defense and Veterans Affairs must now include possible exposure of soldiers to Afghani dogs.

Rabies requires direct inoculation into neural tissue by the infected bite of an infected mammal. The virus infiltrates nerve sheaths and is transmitted to the cells of the CNS. The rapidity of the virus reaching the CNS is a function of the distance from where the bite from the infected animal occurred. Thus the farther from the CNS, the longer the manifestation of symptoms will take to occur.

Human cases are rare in the United States, and rabies stands apart from other viral infections by the long latency period that follows inoculation of the virus with its clinical manifestations. The importance of this disease is that it is fatal once the characteristic clinical features appear, making survival of the individual dependent on quick identification of exposure. Almost all cases of rabies are the result of transdermal viral inoculation by the bite if an animal. Rare cases have been caused by inhalation of the virus shed by bats, as found in those individuals who go caving.[12] Unusual human-to-human transmission has occurred in 2 patients who were recipients of corneal transplants.[3] More commonly cats, wolves, foxes, raccoons, skunks, and other domestic or wild animals are the source of the virus.

Incubation takes about 20 to 60 days or may be as short as 14 days. The incubation time is directly related to the severity of the bite and location relative to the CNS. After the inoculation, the virus replicates in muscle cells and travels to the CNS by sensory and motor nerves by axonal transport. After CNS involvement, the virus is spread rapidly with early selective involvement of the limbic system neurons. Tingling or numbness around the site of the bite even after the wound has healed is characteristic, thought to be the inflammatory response when the virus reaches the sensory ganglion.[12] Main neurologic symptoms occur over 2 to 4 days with fever. Eighty percent of cases are denoted as the furious form, characterized by headache, malaise consistent with apprehension, dysarthria, spasm of the mouth and throat, numbness of the face, diplopia, and facial muscle spasms. Generalized seizures, confusional psychosis, and agitation may follow.

The other, less common form of rabies is known as dumb/paralytic, and comprises about 20% of cases. It is characterized by spinal cord infection with coma gradually following the acute encephalitic symptoms, and death ensues within 4 to 10 days or longer in the paralytic form.[12]

In serum blood studies leukocytosis is found, and albumin is found in the urine. Normal CSF pressure is found, and a lymphocytic pleocytosis is present. Protein count is increased. MRI displays T2 abnormalities in the medial temporal lobes and basal ganglia. Diagnosis is often made from the appearance of symptoms after the bite from a rabid animal. Diagnosis can be made at times by fluorescent antibody staining of corneal smears of skin biopsies from the nape of the neck, although false results have occurred. The presence of rabies antibodies in the CSF is diagnostic. The best diagnosis while the patient is alive is via brain biopsy of the affected animal.

Following a bite from a rabid animal, thorough washing with soap and water, cleaning afterward with benzyl ammonium chloride (Zephiran) has been shown to inactivate the virus.[12] Open wounds also need a tetanus prophylaxis. If a seemingly healthy animal has bitten, a 10-day surveillance time is necessary. If any symptoms of illness appear, the animal must be euthanized and brain tissue sent for appropriate diagnostic tests.

If the animal is found to be rabid, a postexposure prophylaxis should be administered. The human rabies immunoglobulin is administered to affected patient, with half the dose injected into the wound and the other half injected intramuscularly. This treatment provides passive immunization for 10 to 20 days, which allows time for active immunization.[12] Recent progress in vaccine development (human diploid cell vaccine) has decreased the number of doses from 23 to 5, to be given on specific days postexposure (day of exposure and then on days 3, 7, 14, and 28). Moreover, with the advent of the improved vaccine the rate of antibody response and allergic reactions has decreased owing to elimination of the foreign protein.[12]

SUMMARY

Outcomes of meningitis and encephalitis vary according to the etiology, timeliness of diagnosis, and the patient's comorbidities. Patient management, diagnostics, and testing modalities have greatly improved patient outcomes. Because of the public health concern, early attempts at identifying the organism are key, and continued surveillance for these diseases is ongoing. Extremes in climate and seasons will continue to affect the rates of encephalitis. The awareness of the public and preventive efforts of clinicians must be maintained to keep these diagnoses at bay.

REFERENCES

1. Baum S, Koll B. Acute viral meningitis and encephalitis. In: Gorbach S, Bartlett J, Blacklow N, editors. Infectious disease. 3rd edition. Philadelphia: Lippincott, Williams and Wilkins; 2004. p. 1286–91.
2. Cherry J, Bronstein D. Aseptic meningitis and viral meningitis. In: Feigin R, Cherry J, editors. Textbook of Pediatric Infections, vol. 1, 6th edition. Philadelphia: Saunders; Elsevier; 2009. p. 494–9.
3. Jubelt B. Viral infections and postviral syndromes. In: Rowland L, Pedley T, editors. Merritts neurology. 12th edition. Philadelphia: Lippincott Williams & Wilkins; 2010. p. 156–85.
4. Kaplan R. Meningitis and encephalitis. In: Wolfson A, editor. Clinical practice of emergency medicine. 5th edition. Philadelphia: Lippincott, Williams and Wilkins; 2010. p. 884–6.
5. Logan S, MacMahon E. Viral meningitis. BMJ 2008;336:36–40.
6. National Institute of Neurological Disorders and Stroke (2012). Meningitis and encephalitis fact sheet. Retrieved from: http://www.ninds.nih.gov/disorders/encephalitis_meningitis/detail. Accessed September 6, 2012.
7. Solbrig M, Tyler K. Infections of the nervous system, viral infections. In: Bradley W, Daroff R, Fenichel G, editors. Jankovic's neurology in clinical practice. 5th edition. Philadelphia: Elsevier; 2008. p. 1457–87.
8. Kupila L, Vuorinen T, Vainionpaa R, et al. Etiology of aseptic meningitis and encephalitis in an adult population. Neurology 2006;66:75–80.
9. Shalabi M, Whitley RJ. Recurrent benign lymphocytic meningitis. Clin Infect Dis 2006;43:1194–7.
10. Solomon T, Hart I, Beeching N. Viral encephalitis: a clinician's guide. Pract Neurol 2007;7(5):288–305.
11. Tyler K, Adler D. Twenty-eight years of benign recurring Mollaret meningitis. Arch Neurol 1983;40:42–3.
12. Ropper A, Samuels M. Viral infections of the nervous system, Chronic meningitis and prion diseases. In: Roper, Allen & Samuels, Martin, editors. Principals of neurology. 9th edition. New York: McGraw-Hill; 2009. p. 711–45.

13. Tunkel A, Glaser C, Bloch K, et al. The management of encephalitis: clinical practice guidelines by the Infectious Diseases Society of America. Clin Infect Dis 2008;47:303–27.
14. Centers for Disease Control. Information on arboviral encephalitides. 2012. Retrieved from: http://www.cdc.gov/ncidod/dvbid/arbor/arbdet.htm. Accessed September 16, 2012.
15. Centers for Disease Control. Technical fact sheet. Eastern equine encephalitis. 2012. Retrieved from: http://www.cdc.gov/EasterEquineEncephalitis/tech/factSheet.html.
16. Centers for Disease Control: epidemiology & geographic distribution. 2011. Retrieved from: www.cdc.gov/easternequineencephalitis/tech/epi.html#casesbyyear. Accessed September 26, 2012.
17. Western equine encephalitis. Available at: www.gcmad.org/Documents/Western_Equine_Encephalitis.pdf. Accessed September 26, 2012.
18. Centers for Disease Control. 2012 Technical fact sheet. La Crosse encephalitis. Available at: http://www.cdc.gov/lac/tech/fact.html. Accessed September 26, 2012.
19. Centers for Disease Control. West Nile virus disease and other arboviral diseases- United States. 2011. MMWR Morb Mortal Wkly Rep 2011;306:1316–8.
20. Centers for Disease Control: epidemiology & geographic distribution. St Louis encephalitis. 2011. Retrieved from: http://www.cdc.gov/sle/technical/epi.html. Accessed September 26, 2012.
21. Centers for Disease Control. West Nile homepage. Retrieved from: http://www.cdc.gov/nciod/dvbid/westnile/index.htm. Accessed September 6, 2012.
22. Tyler K. Emerging viral infections of the central nervous system. Part 1. Arch Neurol 2009;66(8):939–48.
23. Centers for Disease Control. 2012. Rabies. Retrieved from: http://www.cdc.gov/rabies/resources/news/2011-12-06.html. Accessed November 24, 2012.
24. Centers for Disease Control. Human rabies from exposure to a vampire bat in Mexico. 2011. MMWR Morb Mortal Wkly Rep 2011;60:1050–2.

Brain Abscess

Tess Slazinski, MN, RN, CCRN, CNRN, CCNS

KEYWORDS

- Brain abscess • Intracerebral abscess • Central nervous system infections
- Computed tomography • Magnetic resonance imaging • Aspiration • Excision

KEY POINTS

- Brain abscess is an area of infection within the parenchyma of the brain.
- Formation and maturation of brain abscess typically takes 2 weeks.
- Early recognition of symptoms and modern diagnostic testing have improved the outcomes for brain abscess.

INTRODUCTION

Brain abscess is a focal, intraparenchymal, or meningeal infection that develops into a collection of pus surrounded by a well-circumscribed capsule.[1,2] Brain abscess has been a known complication of otitis media, mastoiditis, frontal or ethmoid sinusitis, dental infections, bacterial endocarditis, and congenital heart defect.[3] This article addresses the pathophysiology, pathogenesis, clinical manifestations, diagnostic criteria, and nursing considerations for patients with a brain abscess.

BACKGROUND

Brain abscess has been traditionally recognized as a central nervous system infection with a poor outcome.[4,5] Patients frequently present with rapid neurologic deterioration, which has contributed to fear of this disease.[5] Modern techniques for brain biopsy, neuroimaging, and laboratory culture analysis have improved the prognosis.[6] In addition, early diagnosis and treatment have improved the outcome of this condition.[6–8]

The prognosis is related to the initial presentation, response to antibiotic therapy, and any systemic conditions or risk factors that may impede immunologic attempts to clear the infection.[5] The mortality rates reported in recent large case series range from 8% to 25%.[6,8–11] According to one author's 10-year data collection on treatment of brain abscess, excision is associated with a better prognosis than aspiration.[6] Poor

Disclosures: None.
Critical Care Nursing Services, Cedars- Sinai Medical Center, 8700 Beverly Boulevard, Los Angeles, CA 90048, USA
E-mail address: tslazin@aol.com

Crit Care Nurs Clin N Am 25 (2013) 381–388
http://dx.doi.org/10.1016/j.ccell.2013.04.001
0899-5885/13/$ – see front matter © 2013 Elsevier Inc. All rights reserved.

prognostic factors include worse functional status at presentation, immunocompromise, and older age.[5]

PATHOPHYSIOLOGY

A brain abscess may occur as a single focus involving contiguous lobes, or as a contiguous, multilobular process.[3] The most common sites of brain abscesses are the frontal and temporal lobes followed, in descending order of frequency, by the frontoparietal, parietal, cerebellar, and occipital lobes. The microorganism enters the brain and produces an initial area of focal cerebritis, which leads to a softening, edema, hyperemia, and petechial hemorrhage.[12] The early lesion (first 1–2 weeks) is poorly demarcated with no evidence of tissue necrosis.[2] After 2 to 3 weeks, fibroblasts from the capillaries adjacent to the focal cerebritis deposit collagen fibers to contain and encapsulate the purulent focus.[2,12–14] The developed abscess consists of 3 layers: a center polymorphonuclear leukocytes and necrosis, a collagenous capsule surrounding the central areas, and peripheral gliosis.[15] A brain abscess acts as an expanding mass lesion and causes edema in the surrounding tissue. The edema may lead to life-threatening complications such as uncal or brainstem herniation, ventricular rupture, ventriculitis, or meningitis.[14]

PATHOGENESIS

Bacteria may invade the brain either by direct spread, which accounts for 20% to 60% of cases, or through hematogenous seeding.[16] The direct spread from a contiguous site usually causes a single brain abscess. Primary infections that can directly spread to the cerebral cortex include subacute and chronic otitis media and mastoiditis (inferior temporal lobe and cerebellum), frontal or ethmoid sinuses (frontal lobe), and dental infection (frontal lobe). Developed countries have seen decreased rates of brain abscess as the result of ear infections.[17,18] Brain abscess arising from a sinus infection remains an important consideration in both adults and children.[19–22] Penetrating trauma to the brain is another direct method of infection. This type of trauma may be the result of any invading foreign body or retained fragments that can result in necrotic tissue and serve as a nidus for infection.[2] In addition, neurosurgical procedures can be a direct source of development of brain abscess.[23–25] The common organisms from direct sources are listed in **Table 1**.

Hematogenous spread via bacteremia is associated with multiple abscesses in the distribution of the middle cerebral artery.[26] Cerebral abscesses usually form at the gray–white matter junction where microinfarction damages the blood-brain barrier.

Table 1
Common organisms from direct sources of brain abscess

Direct Source of Infection	Microorganism
Paranasal sinuses	*Streptococcus* spp, *Haemophilus* spp, *Bacteroides* spp, *Fusobacterium* spp
Odontogenic	*Streptococcus* spp, *Bacteroides* spp, *Prevotella* spp, *Fusobacterium* spp, *Haemophilus* spp
Otogenic	Enterobacteriaceae, *Streptococcus* spp, *Pseudomonas aeruginosa*, *Bacteroides* spp
Penetrating head trauma	*Staphylococcus aureus*, *Enterobacter* spp, *Clostridium* spp
Neurosurgical procedures	*Staphylococcus* spp, *Streptococcus* spp, *Pseudomonas aeruginosa*, *Enterobacter* spp

Conditions that lead to hematogenous seeding of the brain include chronic pulmonary infections, skin infections, pelvic infections, intra-abdominal infections, esophageal dilation, endoscopic sclerosis of esophageal varices, bacterial endocarditis, cyanotic congenital heart diseases, and intrapulmonary right-to-left shunting in patients with arteriovenous malformations.[27–31] The common organisms from hematogenous seeding are listed in **Table 2**.

CLINICAL MANIFESTATIONS

The clinical manifestations of brain abscess may be nonspecific, which results in a delay in establishing the diagnosis. The diagnosis is made at an average of 13 to 14 days after the onset of symptoms.[2] Unfortunately, fever, which is usually a reliable indicator of infection, occurs in only 50% of patients with a brain abscess.[12,32]

The most common symptom is headache, which is often localized to the side of the abscess. Headache onset may be sudden or gradual. The pain tends to be severe and usually not relieved with over-the-counter remedies. Nuchal rigidity occurs in 15% of patients with brain abscess and is most commonly associated with occipital-lobe abscess or an abscess that has ruptured into the subarachnoid space.[12] If the abscess ruptures into the subarachnoid space, the headache is sudden and severe.

Focal neurologic deficits occur in 50% of patients and occur days to weeks after the onset of headache.[32] The deficit depends on location of the brain abscess. Neurologic deficits from temporal-lobe involvement may include Wernicke aphasia, contralateral facial droop, and homonymous superior quandranopsia. Patients with frontal-lobe lesions may have drowsiness, impaired judgment, seizures, and/or contralateral hemiparesis. Parietal-lobe lesions may lead to patients presenting with homonymous hemianopsia, and impaired proprioception and stereoagnosis. Cerebellar abscess may manifest as ataxia and nystagmus. Patients with abscesses that involve the brainstem may present with multiple cranial nerve findings and contralateral hemiparesis.

As the abscess increases in size, patients may display signs of increased intracranial pressure. Clinical manifestations for patients may include decreased level of consciousness, vomiting, palsies of cranial nerves III and VI, and/or papilledema. These manifestations can lead to catastrophic complications such as uncal or brainstem herniation.

DIAGNOSIS

Computed tomography (CT) is performed for emergency cases. When a brain abscess is suspected, the study must be performed with a contrast agent. The lesion has different appearances based on the age of the abscess.[13] Early cerebritis appears as an irregular area of low density that does not enhance following contrast injection.

Table 2 Common organisms from hematogenous seeding	
Hematogenous Infection Source	**Microorganism**
Lungs	*Streptococcus* spp, *Fusobacterium* spp, *Actinomyces* spp
Urinary tract	*Pseudomonas aeruginosa*, *Enterobacter* spp
Endocarditis	Viridans streptococci, *Staphylococcus aureus*
Congenital cardiac malformations (especially right-to-left shunts)	*Streptococcus* spp

As cerebritis evolves, the lesion enlarges with thick and diffuse ring enhancement following contrast injection. The ring contrast enhancement represents breakdown of the blood-brain barrier and development of an inflammatory capsule.

Magnetic resonance imaging (MRI) is the preferred study. MRI should be performed with gadolinium, which increases the T1 intensity and causes more prominent enhancement of lesions than a CT scan. In addition, MRI is preferred over CT because it is more sensitive for early cerebritis and in detecting satellite lesions; more accurately estimates the extent of central necrosis, ring enhancement, and cerebral edema; and provides better visualization of the brainstem. Diffusion-weighted MRI is capable of differentiating ring-enhancing lesions caused by a brain abscess from neoplastic lesions.[33,34]

Laboratory specimens obtained from stereotactic CT-guided aspiration or surgery should be sent for Gram stain, and aerobic, anaerobic, mycobacterial, and fungal culture. In addition, special stains including an acid-fast stain for mycobacteria, modified acid-fast stain for *Nocardia*, and fungal stains should be performed to aid in the identification of the etiologic agent.[2] Serology specimens may aid in the diagnosis of *Toxoplasma gondii* or neurocysticercosis infections. Anti-*Toxoplasma* immunoglobulin G antibody may be present in blood, and anticysticercal antibodies on cerebrospinal fluid specimens.[2] Current literature has demonstrated promising results from 16S ribosomal sequencing studies. Amplification of 16S ribosomal DNA by polymerase chain reaction increased the number of bacterial species isolated from brain abscesses in comparison with standard culture. According to the investigators, several new species were identified.[35–37]

TREATMENT

The clinical manifestations of brain abscess can be subtle, which may lead to a delay in treatment. There must be an index of suspicion for central nervous system infection. The treatment usually requires a combination of antibiotics, glucocorticoids (dexamethasone), and surgical drainage.[8,38] The usual course of antibiotic therapy is 4 to 8 weeks. Medications, dosage, and indications are summarized in **Table 3**.

The neurosurgery service needs to be consulted at the time of initial diagnosis of brain abscess. Needle aspiration and surgical excision have both been used to treat brain abscess. Needle aspiration is performed by placing a burr hole, then inserting the needle under CT guidance. The aspirate needs to be cultured for aerobes and anaerobes, fungi, and *Mycobacterium tuberculosis*.[39] Brain abscesses should be reaspirated if they fail to change in size or expand in diameter.[39] Stereotactic guidance has improved the precision of needle aspiration, and is preferred for lesions that involve the speech areas and motor and sensory cortices.[40] It is also the preferred method for comatose patients.[40]

Surgical excision is not performed as often as needle aspiration, because of a greater risk for neurologic complications. Excision may be the treatment of choice for the following situations: traumatic brain abscess (to remove bone chips and foreign material), encapsulated fungal brain abscesses, and multiloculated abscesses.[39] Surgical excision may be necessary after aspiration when the following occur: no clinical improvement within 1 week, signs of increased intracranial pressure, and increased abscess ring diameter.[39]

NURSING CONSIDERATIONS

Critical care nurses, who care for critically ill patients, are vital members of the health care team. Nurses play a significant role in decreasing the complications associated

Table 3
Summary of antibiotic therapy for brain abscess

Drug name	Dosage	Indication
Metronidazole	15 mg/kg IV loading dose, followed by 7.5 mg/kg IV every eight hours; not to exceed 4 g/day	Brain abscesses arising from oral, otogenic, or sinus source (ie, chronic otitis or mastoiditis, where the site of abscess is usually the temporal lobe or cerebellum; or frontal or ethmoid sinusitis, where the site of abscess is usually the frontal lobe)
Penicillin G	20 to 24 million units per day IV in six equally divided doses	Administered in combination with Metronidazole, especially for oral focus
Ceftriaxone	2 g IV every twelve hours	
Cefotaxime	2 g IV every four to six hours	OR
		Ceftriaxone and Metronidazole
		OR
		Cefotaxime and Metronidazole
Vancomycin	30 mg/kg IV daily in two equally divided doses adjusted for renal function	Brain abscess from hematogenous spread
Nafcillin	2 g IV every four hours	Nafcillin or oxacillin would replace Vancomycin when susceptibility
Oxacillin	2 g IV every four hours	testing reveals methicillin-sensitive *S Aureus*
Vancomycin	30 mg/kg IV daily in two equally divided doses adjusted for renal function	Postoperative neurosurgical patients Vancomycin and ceftazidime OR
Ceftazidime	2 g IV every eight hours	Vancomycin and cefepime
Cefepime	2 g IV every eight hours	OR
Meropenem	1 g IV every eight hours	Vancomycin and meropenem
Nafcillin	2 g IV every four hours	Nafcillin or oxacillin would replace
Oxacillin	2 g IV every four hours	Vancomycin when susceptibility testing reveals methicillin-sensitive *S Aureus*
Vancomycin	30 mg/kg IV daily in two equally divided doses adjusted for renal function	Brain abscess following penetrating trauma Vancomycin and ceftriaxone
Ceftriaxone	2 g IV every twelve hours	OR
Cefotaxime	2 g IV every four to six hours	Vancomycin and cefotaxime
Nafcillin	2 g IV every four hours	Nafcillin or oxacillin would replace
Oxacillin	2 g IV every four hours	Vancomycin when susceptibility testing reveals methicillin-sensitive *S Aureus*

Abbreviation: IV, intravenous.

with this group of patients. A baseline neurologic examination and serial neurologic assessment assist in early recognition of findings that indicate increased intracranial pressure from an expanding lesion, cerebral edema, or abscess rupture.[3] The frequency of the neurologic assessment depends on the severity of the patient's condition. Components of the neurologic examination that may demonstrate neurologic decline are level of consciousness, motor examination, and cranial nerves. In addition, examination of meningeal irritation may indicate abscess rupture or subarachnoid hemorrhage. Nuchal rigidity, and Brudzinski and Kernig signs are important factors to include in the serial neurologic examination, as these are signs of meningeal irritation.

The critical care nurse is responsible for the safe, timely administration of antibiotics.[3,30] Drug compatibilities, drug interactions, and drug toxicity (nephrotoxicity and heptatotoxicity) must be important considerations for nurses. If necessary, consultation with nurse case managers for in-home intravenous therapy is an essential component of discharge planning.[3] Patients also need to receive education regarding their medication regime, signs and symptoms to be monitored, and follow-up appointments to be honored.[30]

Critical care nurses play an important role in the prevention of nosocomial infection. Hand washing and donning personal protective equipment are the most effective ways to prevent the spread of infection, especially in immunocompromised and chronically ill patients. In addition, nurses ensure that proper hand washing is performed by all health care providers and family members before they enter and after they exit the patient's room.

REFERENCES

1. Sarmast AF, Showkat JI, Kirmani AR, et al. Aspiration versus excision: a single center experience of forty-seven patients with brain abscess over 10 years. Neurol Med Chir 2012;52:724–30.
2. Southwick F. Pathogenesis, clinical manifestations, and diagnosis of brain abscess. Available at: www.UpToDate.com. Accessed October 2012.
3. Twomey CR. Brain abscess: an update. J Neurosci Nurs 1992;24(1):34–9.
4. Wing S. Brain abscess. J Neurosurg Nurs 1981;13(3):123–6.
5. Heth JA. Neurosurgical aspects of central nervous system infections. Neuroimaging Clin N Am 2012;22:791–9.
6. Sarmast AH, Showkat HI, Bhat AR, et al. Analysis and management of brain abscess; a ten-year hospital based study. Turk Neurosurg 2012;22(6):682–9.
7. Tseng MY. Brain abscess in 142 patients: factors influencing outcome and mortality. Surg Neurol 2006;65(6):557–62.
8. Cavusoglu H, Kaya RA, Turkmenoglu ON, et al. Brain abscess: analysis of results in a series of 51 patients with a combined surgical and medical approach during an 11-year period. Neurosurg Focus 2008;24(6):E9.
9. Auvichayapat N, Auvichayapat P, Augwarawong S. Brain abscess in infants and children: a retrospective study of 107 patients in Northeast Thailand. J Med Assoc Thai 2007;90:1601–7.
10. Carpenter J, Stapleton S, Hollman R. Retrospective analysis of 49 cases of brain abscess and review of the literature. Eur J Clin Microbiol Infect Dis 2007;26: 1–11.
11. Prasad KN, Mishra AM, Gupta D. Analysis of microbial etiology and mortality in patients with brain abscess. J Infect 2006;53:221–7.
12. McKinney AS. Brain abscess. Hosp Med 1983;19:13–21.
13. Britt RH, Enzman DR. Clinical stages of human brain abscesses on serial CT scans after contrast infusion: computerized tomographic, neuropathological, and clinical correlations. J Neurosurg 1983;59:972–89.
14. Tunkel AR. Brain abscess. In: Mandell GL, Bennett JE, Dolin R, editors. Mandell, Douglas, and Bennett's principles and practice of infectious diseases. 7th edition. Philadelphia: Churchill, Livingstone, and Elsevier; 2010. p. 1265–79.
15. Carey ME, Chou MB, French LA. Experience with brain abscess. J Neurosurg 1983;3(6):272–4.

16. Chun CH, Johnson JD, Hofstetter M, et al. Brain abscess: a study of 45 consecutive cases. Medicine (Baltimore) 1986;65:415–31.
17. Kangsanarak J, Fooanant S, Ruchphaopunt K, et al. Extracranial and intracranial complications of suppurative otitis media. Report of 102 cases. J Laryngol Otol 1993;107:999–1004.
18. Yen PT, Chan ST, Huang TS. Brain abscess: with special reference to otolaryngologic sources of infection. Otolaryngol Head Neck Surg 1995;113:15–22.
19. Chalstrey S, Pfeiderer AG, Moffat DA. Persisting incidence and mortality of sinogenic cerebral abscess: a continuing reflection of late clinical diagnosis. J R Soc Med 1991;84:193–5.
20. Giannoni CM, Stewart MG, Alford EL. Intracranial complications of sinusitis. Laryngoscope 1997;107:863–7.
21. Giannoni CM, Sulek M, Friedman EM. Intracranial complications of sinusitis: a pediatric series. Am J Rhinol 1998;12:173–8.
22. Gallagher RM, Gross CW, Phillips CD. Suppurative intracranial complications of sinusitis. Laryngoscope 1998;108:1635–42.
23. Henao-Martinez AF, Young H, Nardi-Korver JJ, et al. *Mycoplasma hominis* brain abscess presenting after a head trauma: a case report. J Med Case Rep 2012; 6:253.
24. Morton R, Lucas TH, Ko A. Intracerebral abscess associated with the Camino intracranial pressure monitor: case report and review of the literature. Neurosurgery 2012;71(1):E193–8.
25. Staecker H, Nadol JB Jr, Ojeman R, et al. Delayed intracranial abscess after acoustic neuroma surgery: a report of two cases. Am J Otol 1999;20(3): 293–408.
26. Bakski R, Wright PD, Kinkel PR, et al. Cranial magnetic resonance imaging findings in bacterial endocarditis: the neuroimaging spectrum of septic brain embolization demonstrated in twelve patients. J Neuroimaging 1999;9:78–84.
27. Schlaffer F, Riesenberg K, Mikolich D, et al. Serious bacterial infections after endoscopic procedures. Arch Intern Med 1996;156:572–4.
28. Takeshita M, Kagawa M, Yato S, et al. Current treatment of brain abscess in patients with congenital cyanotic heart disease. Neurosurgery 1997;41:1270–9.
29. Cahill DP, Barker FG, Davis KR, et al. Case records of the Massachusetts General Hospital. Case 10-2010. A 37 year old woman with weakness and a mass in the brain. N Engl J Med 2010;362:1326–33.
30. Gulek BG, Rapport R. Infectious intracranial aneurysms: triage and management. J Neurosci Nurs 2011;43(1):51–6.
31. Tamarit M, Poveda P, Baron M, et al. Four cases of nocardial brain abscess. Surg Neurol Int 2012;3:88.
32. Seydoux C, Francioli P. Bacterial brain abscesses: factors influencing mortality and sequelae. Clin Infect Dis 1992;15:394–401.
33. Leuthardt EC, Wippold FJ 2nd, Oswood MC, et al. Diffusion-weighted MR imaging in the preoperative assessment of brain abscesses. Surg Neurol 2002;58(6): 395–402.
34. Friedlander RM, Gonzalez RG, Afridi NA, et al. Case records of the Massachusetts General Hospital. Weekly clinicopathological exercises. Case 16-2003. A 58 year old woman with left-sided weakness and a right frontal brain mass. N Engl J Med 2003;348(21):2125–32.
35. Raoultm D, Al Masalma M, Armougom F, et al. The expansion of the microbiological spectrum of brain abscesses with use of multiple 16S ribosomal DNA sequencing. Clin Infect Dis 2009;48(9):1169–78.

36. Keller PM, Rampini SK, Bloemberg GV, et al. Detection of a mixed infection in a culture-negative brain abscess by broad-spectrum bacterial 16S rRNA gene PCR. J Clin Microbiol 2010;48(6):2250–2.

37. Al Masalma M, Lonjon M, Ricket H, et al. Metagenomic analysis of brain abscesses identifies specific bacterial associations. Clin Infect Dis 2012;54(2): 202–10.

38. Arlotti M, Grossi P, Pea F, et al. Consensus document on controversial issues for the treatment of infections of the central nervous system: bacterial brain abscesses. Int J Infect Dis 2010;14(Suppl 4):S79–92.

39. Southwick FS. Treatment and prognosis of brain abscess. Available at: www. UpToDate.com. Accessed October 2012.

40. Ratnaike TE, Das S, Gregson BA, et al. A review of brain abscess surgical treatment—78 years: aspiration versus excision. World Neurosurg 2011;76(5):431–6.

Spinal Epidural Abscess

Katherine G. Johnson, MS, CNS-BC, CCRN, CNRN

KEYWORDS

- Spinal abscess • Spinal epidural abscess • Back pain • Spinal cord compression
- Spinal infection

KEY POINTS

- Spinal abscess is an area of infection within the epidural space of the spinal canal.
- Early diagnosis of back pain is important before symptoms of spinal cord compression develop.
- Treatment includes antibiotics and possibly surgical drainage of the abscess.
- Most patients recover with no neurologic deficits.

INTRODUCTION

Infections of the spine are rare and present with a variety of nonspecific signs and symptoms, making them a diagnostic challenge. Infections of the spine include osteomyelitis and epidural, subdural, and intradural abscesses.[1] Specifically, a spinal epidural abscess (SEA) is a localized bacterial infection above the dural layer of the spinal meninges.

SEA is most often located in the thoracic[2] and lumbar spinal regions.[3] Onset of symptoms may be sudden or slowly progressive and can be the result of systemic bacteremia or septicemia. The most common causative organism is *Staphylococcus aureus*. Favorable outcome requires prompt diagnosis,[4] early medical, and often surgical interventions to prevent the development of neurologic deficits[5,6] or even death.[3,7,8] Nurses play an important role in caring for patients with SEA, from the early phases of diagnosis and treatment to the later phases of recovery and rehabilitation.[4,9]

EPIDEMIOLOGY

Spinal epidural abscesses are relatively uncommon, 2 to 3 per 10,000 hospital admissions.[5,10] Although rare, a rising incidence over the last 2 decades may be attributed to an aging population, a rise in the number of invasive spinal procedures, and an increase in intravenous drug use.[5] Other potential explanations for the increase are related to predisposing conditions, such as diabetes mellitus, alcoholism, or HIV infections.[5]

Disclosures: None.
Patient Care Consulting Services, The Queens Medical Center, 1301 Punchbowl Street, Honolulu, HI 96813, USA
E-mail address: kjohnson@queens.org

Crit Care Nurs Clin N Am 25 (2013) 389–397
http://dx.doi.org/10.1016/j.ccell.2013.04.002
0899-5885/13/$ – see front matter © 2013 Elsevier Inc. All rights reserved.

SEA occurs in all age groups, with a greater incidence in those between the ages of 50 and 70, and slightly more men than women.[6,10] IV drug users who develop an SEA are commonly younger than 50.[11] Men are also more likely to have primary rather than secondary SEA.[12] The thoracic level is the most common site for an SEA in 50% to 80% of the cases, less commonly the lumbar region (17%–38%), followed by the lumbar and cervical sites (10%–25%).[11] SEA is rarely diagnosed in children.[12]

PREDISPOSING CONDITIONS

SEA is associated with systemic states of altered immune function, such as diabetes mellitus, end-stage renal disease, septicemia, immunocompromised states, malignancy, morbid obesity, or alcoholism. Discitis or vertebral osteomyelitis is associated findings in 80% to 100% of patients.[11] Local factors that contribute to the development of SEA include spinal trauma, spinal surgery, and intrathecal injection or catheter placement into the vertebral canal.[13] A history of spinal trauma accounts for 10% to 30% of cases.[11]

Patients that develop SEA usually have one or more comorbidities. The most common comorbidity is an underlying infectious process. Primary SEA is diagnosed when bacteria gain access to the epidural space through contiguous spread (primary) or hematogenous dissemination[5,12] from elsewhere in the body, such as skin lesions or oral foci. The abscess can be located in either the anterior or the posterior epidural space.[2] Secondary SEA, a type of surgical site infection, occurs after direct introduction of pathogens into the epidural space.[12,13] This infection may occur after spinal trauma, injections, surgery, or during lumbar punctures or epidural analgesia. In a 4-year prospective study of 36 patients, primary SEA was found in 44% of patients and was secondary to elective spinal procedures in 56%.[12]

DIAGNOSIS

Diagnosis of SEA is based on clinical presentation and supported by laboratory and imaging data. Diagnosis may be delayed when there is no characteristic clinical presentation, and radiographs are frequently noninformative.[14] The first published case of SEA was reported in the literature in 1761, describing a 40-year-old man who presented with severe pain and paralysis of the lower extremities.[6]

Clinical Presentation

The diagnosis of SEA may be difficult and delayed because early signs and symptoms may be difficult to distinguish from other causes of back or neck pain. A 4-stage progression of SEA signs and symptoms was introduced in 1948.[3] The first phase presents as nonspecific clinical symptoms, such as back pain, fever, and malaise. The second phase is characterized by radiculopathy and paresthesias. Symptoms commonly seen in the third phase include motor and sensory deficits and bowel or bladder dysfunction. Last, 34% of patients will present in the final stage, paralysis.[3,6] Average time from back pain to nerve root symptoms is 3 days; 4.5 days from nerve root symptoms to weakness, and 24 hours from weakness to paraplegia.[15]

For most patients, the classic symptom triad of fever, back pain, and neurologic deficits may be absent, and, if present, may indicate a progression to irreversible symptoms.[7] A meta-analysis of 915 patients revealed that fever was present in 66%, back pain in 71%, and muscle weakness in 26% of SEA patients.[6] Fever is frequently absent in patients with a history of intravenous drug usage.[1]

Davis and colleagues[7] analyzed 1019 patients seen in their emergency department with back or neck pain. Their primary goal was to determine the incidence of diagnostic delay and motor deficits before and after the implementation of a decision guideline to screen patients for SEA in the emergency department patient. Their guideline includes assessments such as pain, progressive neurologic deficits, fever, risk factors, and causes of symptoms, followed by inflammatory markers before magnetic resonance imaging (MRI) evaluation. They reported a statistically significant reduction in diagnostic delay after implementation of their guideline. They noted that a risk factor was present in 100% of the 86 patients that were diagnosed with SEA. Most commonly were IV drug abuse, other sites of infection, or recent spinal procedures. Only 2% of patients had the classic triad of fever, pain, and neurologic deficit at initial presentation. They concluded that their treatment guideline, incorporating risk factor assessment followed by C-reactive protein (CRP) and erythrocyte sedimentation rate (ESR) testing, was highly sensitive and moderately specific for identifying SEA in an emergency department patient. In addition, the guideline was shown to prevent diagnostic delays. These guidelines may assist in the early diagnosis of patients with SEA when neurologic symptoms may be vague or not apparent.

Laboratory

Inflammatory markers, such as white blood cell count, CRP, and ESR, are worth evaluating. Leukocytosis is found in 60% to 80% of acute cases and ESR greater than 20 mm/h is found in up to 95% of cases.[3] White blood cell count may be normal for chronic cases.[10] The most common bacterial pathogen, S aureus,[5] occurs in 60% to 90% of cases. An increasing incidence is noted in methicillin-resistant Staphylococcus aureus.

Imaging

MRI scanning is currently the diagnostic standard.[2,14] Gadolinium-enhanced MRI is the most sensitive, specific, and accurate imaging method[3] that is also useful in distinguishing epidural abscess from other potential compressive lesions. When an SEA is present, MR images reveal a T1 hypo-intense, T2 hyperintense mass in the epidural space.[2] A computed tomographic (CT) scan does not always provide conclusive evidence of SEA[12]; however, a CT with myelography may be considered if an MRI is unavailable or contraindicated.[11]

Microbiological Studies

It is important to cultivate the causative organism from blood or from the abscess itself. Bacteremia causing or arising from spinal epidural abscess is detected in about 60% of patients.[10] Cultures from blood and other possible sources of infection, such as septic emboli, and potential aerobic, anaerobic, mycobacterial, and fungal organisms are recommended. A CT-guided needle aspiration of the abscess may be performed because blood cultures have been found to be negative in 40% of cases.[3]

The most common causative organism, S aureus, is present in 50% to 70% of cases.[6,10,12] This S aureus is followed by aerobic and anaerobic streptococcus species in 7% of the cases. Gram-negative bacteria may be more commonly found in IV drug users[1] or in non-Western countries.[16] Fungal infections may be seen in immunocompromised patients and SEA because parasitic organisms may be seen in certain geographic regions.[6] Patients with multiple comorbidities may present with several organisms.[12]

Surgical Consult

Surgical interventions are the treatment of choice for most patients.[3] Urgent decompressive surgery is indicated to control sepsis and minimize neurologic damage. An infectious disease specialist may be needed to assist in the optimal selection of antimicrobial agents.[11]

TREATMENT

Bacterial SEA is considered to be an emergency.[17] The goals include eradication of the microorganism and drainage of the abscess.[3] Medical, surgical, or combinations of management should be the treatment of choice[5] and determined with multidisciplinary involvement from spine surgeons, infectious disease specialists, radiologists, and pharmacists.

Pharmacologic

The choice of antibiotic depends on the suspected source of infection. Antibiotic coverage should begin as soon as cultures from potential sources of infection have been obtained.[3] Empiric antibiotic therapy should include coverage for anti-Staphylococcus organisms, as well antimicrobial coverage against streptococci and gram-negative bacilli. Once the causative organism is identified, antibiotic treatment can be adjusted accordingly. Typically, vancomycin along with ceftazidime or cefepime[5] and metronidazole would be offered.

There are no definitive treatment durations for intravenous or subsequent oral regimens. Generally, resolution of the abscess is achieved after 4 to 6 weeks of therapy; however, those with vertebral osteomyelitis may require up to 8 to 12 weeks.[3] Treatment is based on comorbidities, type of treatment provided, microorganism identified, and bacterial effect of the available agent.[3] Treatment success is confirmed by follow-up imaging studies 4 to 8 weeks after therapy.[3]

Surgical Intervention

The surgical management of infections corresponds to the location and degree of spinal cord compression.[18] Most patients with SEA will undergo prompt decompressive surgery to prevent permanent disability. Surgical intervention allows for cord decompression, removal of devitalized tissue, and drainage and irrigation of the abscess. An abscess can be easily removed if encapsulated or aspirated when there are no walls.[17] A tissue drain may be left in place postoperatively to allow for irrigation and installation of fluids or medications.

A hemi-laminectomy at one or more levels can be performed to drain an abscess posterior to the dura. More extensive infections may involve fusions or instrumentation to provide stabilization. Immobilization with a halo-vest for cervical infections or a thoracolumbar sacral orthosis for thoracic through sacral infections is a treatment option.[15]

CT-Guided Needle Aspiration

A CT-guided needle aspiration is a diagnostic procedure that may also have therapeutic benefits by reducing the size of the inflammation. Candidates for this procedure are patients with a posterior SEA, neurologically intact patients, high-risk surgical patients, or those unresponsive to antimicrobial treatment alone.[3] This minimally invasive needle aspiration may be performed through the sacral canal using CT fluoroscopic guidance. Aspiration of the abscess followed by intravenous antibiotics may be an effective alternative to a surgical procedure.[19] After needle aspiration of the abscess, frequent neurologic assessments are required to monitor for incomplete drainage or spinal canal compromise.[11] Post procedure patient education focuses on recognizing neurologic deterioration, signs and symptoms of infection, and care of the incision.

Conservative Therapy

Conservative options alone might be used to control the infection for specific indications. Patients with prohibitive operative risk factors, involvement of an extensive length of the spinal canal, complete paresis for more than 3 days,[3,15] or those with a presumed lack of benefit may be offered nonsurgical conservative management alone. A trial of serial neurologic evaluations, spinal MRIs, and antibiotics may be used in an attempt to avoid surgical intervention.[11]

In a retrospective chart review of 48 patients conducted by Curry and colleagues,[10] 48% of their SEA patients who lacked neurologic deficits were offered antibiotic therapy alone as the initial treatment strategy. Fifty-two percent of these conservatively treated patients worsened and only 13% improved. Their data suggested that improved outcomes in SEA are more readily achieved via urgent surgery rather than a conservative nonoperative approach.

However, Karikari and colleagues[20] do not support the hypothesis that patients treated without early surgery are more likely to have a poor outcome. They reviewed 104 patients managed nonoperatively and report that 64% of their patients remained stable and 11% improved. They also found that patients with ventral SEA may be more likely to be successfully treated conservatively as opposed to those with a dorsal SEA.

Because of the potential for rapid deterioration, the status of patients treated nonsurgically must be monitored very closely. Frequent follow-up examinations and laboratory and imaging studies should be conducted.[3] With frequent monitoring, patients who are treated conservatively can have an uneventful recovery.

OUTCOMES

Outcome is largely determined by the extent and duration of preoperative neurologic deficits.[5,10] Therefore, since 1923, surgical decompression combined with antibiotics is the treatment of choice for SEA.[6] Factors crucial for the assessment of outcome are mortality and recovery from neurologic deficits.[3] Factors that affect prognosis include a delay in diagnosis or evaluation, the development of significant paresis or paralysis before or during treatment, or an immune-compromised state.[11] Duration of symptoms have an impact on outcomes. Darouiche[5] noted an improvement in muscle power in 86% of paralyzed patients who underwent surgery within 24 hours. Wang and colleagues[1] found that patients in their study that presented with motor deficits of less than 3 days had significant improvement with surgery and only 2 of 12 patients showed significant improvement when their deficit was greater than 3 days.

According to Chao and Nanda,[21] surgery provides a good outcome when patients' spinal cord symptoms are present for fewer than 72 hours, when extent of the abscess (the degree of thecal sac compression) is less than 50%, and when patients are younger than 60 years of age. Improved outcomes in SEA are also more readily achieved via urgent surgery rather than with a conservative, nonoperative approach.[10] However, despite more sophisticated diagnostic options and heightened awareness, outcomes of an SEA remain poor, with only about 45% of patients achieving a full recovery[10] and mortality remaining as high as 23%.[20] During the disease course, elevated CRP levels in the second week after admission can also be a prognostic indicator.[3] Follow-up MRIs and neurologic examinations are necessary to ensure adequate treatment and resolution of symptoms.

ACUTE AND POSTOPERATIVE NURSING CARE

Nursing management of a patient with an SEA depends on the treatment required, neurologic deficits, and spinal stability. A variety of interventions are individualized to the patient's degree of deficits and treatment regime (**Box 1**). Expected patient outcomes include fall prevention, knowledge of the disease process and treatment regimen,[18] and promotion of self-management strategies. The nurse's primary goal during the postoperative period is preventing neurologic deterioration through early detection of changes and timely interventions. The nurse coordinates a collaborative team to maintain pain control, foster adherence to the treatment regimen, minimize complications, enhance mobility, and coordinate rehabilitation and discharge needs.

Neurologic Assessments

Assessments begin on admission and should provide baseline data about functional status, level of the lesion, and other associated problems.[18] Frequent monitoring for potential deterioration, motor strength, and sensory abnormalities; mental status; and onset of increased muscle tone or persistent numbness are standard interventions.[22] The frequency and intensity will vary based on the patient's level of deficit and treatment offered. Increased frequency of monitoring is encouraged if neurologic deterioration is detected.

Pain Management

A comprehensive pain assessment is helpful to assess for location, characteristics, onset, duration, frequency, intensity, severity, and precipitating factors.[22] Knowledge of the patient's current use of preoperative pharmacologic and nonpharmacologic methods of pain relief will be beneficial in facilitating postoperative pain management approaches. Pharmacologic and nonpharmacologic measures should be provided for

---

Box 1
Potential nursing interventions

- Activity therapy
- Anxiety reduction
- Behavior management
- Caregiver support
- Coping enhancement
- Fall prevention
- Infection protection
- Medication management
- Neurologic assessments
- Nutrition management
- Pain management
- Peripheral sensation management
- Prevention of complications from immobility
- Positioning, neurologic
- Positioning, wheelchair
- Teaching disease process
- Urinary elimination management

Data from Refs.[9,21,22]

pain control. Nurses need to assess patient's pain and intervention effectiveness continually.

Positioning and Mobility

Impaired mobility related to the neurologic deficit or postoperative phase should be anticipated. Mobilization should be customized to the patient's activity level. Proper neurologic positioning and appropriate body alignment for the patient at risk for spinal cord injury or vertebral irritability may be achieved with immobilizing devices such as halos or cervical collars. Some patients may also require a wheelchair to enhance comfort and foster independence.[22] Due to possible immobility, deep vein thrombosis prophylaxis is another intervention that should be implemented. Patients will be free of immobility complications when nursing has provided appropriate interventions.

Infection

Most all SEA patients will have a bacterial infection. Rapid identification of the bacterial organism will require prompt interventions related to obtaining specimens and responding to laboratory results. Prevention of the spread of a nosocomial infection is important during all phases of care and recovery, including in the operating room.[22] Nursing activities such as monitoring for systemic and localized signs of infection, such as incision wound healing, will be necessary. Administration of antimicrobial agents and reinforcement of outpatient medication regimens are strongly encouraged. Patients should be taught the importance of proper hand hygiene, signs and symptoms of infection, and maintenance of long-term intravenous access.[23]

Patient Education

Assisting the patient to understand information related to their disease process is a vital nursing activity.[22] Explanations of the pathophysiology of the disease and the patient's current knowledge of their risk factors are important teaching points. For patients with SEA, comorbidities and social situations may need to be addressed if they are contributing to illness or hindering recovery.

Self-Management Strategies

Neurologic deterioration may leave a patient with partial or total self-care deficits. Activities that encourage independence with ADLs are beneficial. Some patients may require bowel or bladder elimination management.

Rehabilitation

Rehabilitation programs are advised for patients with neurologic deficits or diminished mobility. Rehabilitation specialists can assist with progressive strengthening and progressive mobility and move the patient toward increasing independence with ADLs. Collaboration with occupational, physical, and/or recreational therapists is helpful to optimize the patient's postoperative activity level or adjustment to disabilities. Therapy to improve strength and gait is often needed, and the rate of recovery may be slow.[11]

SUMMARY

Early diagnosis and treatment of SEA result in lower rates of long-term disability. Patients with localized back pain, particularly those with fever and other risk factors, should undergo an immediate MRI study to ensure early diagnosis and management. Treatment typically consists of antibiotics, immobilization, and potential surgical intervention. Patient outcomes are likely to be favorable if treatment is initiated before the development of neurologic signs and symptoms. Providing appropriate nursing assessments and interventions will assist the patient in achieving the best possible outcomes.

REFERENCES

1. Wang Z, Lenehan B, Itshayek E, et al. Primary pyogenic infection of the spine in intravenous drug users. Spine 2012;37:685–92.
2. Diehn F. Imaging of spine infection. Radiol Clin North Am 2012;50:777–98.
3. Sendi P, Bregenzer T, Zimmerli W. Spinal epidural abscess in clinical practice. QJM 2008;101:1–12.
4. Alvarez M. SEA - from onset to rehabilitation: case study. J Neurosci Nurs 2005; 37(2):72–7.
5. Darouiche R. Spinal epidural abscess. N Engl J Med 2006;355:2012–20.
6. Reihsaus E, Waldbaur H, Seeling W. Spinal epidural abscess; a meta-analysis of 915 patients. Neurosurg Rev 2000;232:175–204.
7. Davis D, Salazar A, Chan T, et al. Progressive evaluation of clinical decision guideline to diagnose spinal epidural abscess in patients who present to the emergency department with spine pain. J Neurosurg Spine 2011;14:765–70.
8. Deshmukh V. Midline corpectomies for the evacuation of an extensive ventral cervical and upper thoracic spinal epidural abscess. J Neurosurg Spine 2010;13: 229–33.
9. Gilliland K. Epidural abscess of the spine: case comparisons. J Neurosci Nurs 1989;21(3):185–9.
10. Curry W, Hoh B, Amin-Hanjani S, et al. Spinal epidural abscess: clinical presentation, management, and outcome. Surg Neurol 2005;63:364–71.
11. Spinal Epidural Abscess 2012. eResource. In Medical Topics: First Consult. Available at: http://www.firstconsult.com/das/pdxmd/body/395311825-37/1399204971?type= med&eid=9-u1.0-_1_mt_1011036. Accessed September 14, 2012.
12. Zimmerer S, Conen A, Muller A, et al. Spinal epidural abscess: aetiology, predisponent factors and clinical outcomes in a 4 year prospective study, 2011 factors and clinical outcomes in a 4 year prospective study. Eur Spine J 2011;20: 2228–34.
13. Tompkins M, Panuncialman I, Lucas P, et al. Spinal epidural abscess. J Emerg Med 2010;39:384–90.
14. Urrutia J, Rojas C. Extensive epidural abscess with surgical treatment and long term follow up. Spine J 2007;7:708–11.
15. Greenberg M. Handbook of neurosurgery. 6th edition. New York: Thieme; 2006. p. 240–3.
16. Huang C, Lu C, Chuang Y, et al. Clinical characteristics and therapeutic outcome of gram-negative bacterial spinal epidural abscess in adults. J Clin Neurosci 2011;18:213–7.
17. Priutt A. Neurologic infections disease emergencies. Neurol Clin 2012;30: 129–59.
18. Miers A. Nontraumatic disorders of the Spine. In: Barker E, editor. Neuroscience nursing a spectrum of care. 3rd edition. St. Louis, MO: Mosby; 2008. p. 436–71.
19. Kostanian VT, Mathews MS. Minimally invasive approach for drainage of a sacral epidural abscess. Interv Neuroradiol 2007;13:161–5.
20. Karikari I, Powers C, Reynolds R, et al. Management of spontaneous spinal epidural abscess: a single-center 10 year experience. Neurosurgery 2009;65: 919–24.

21. Chao D, Nanda A. Spinal epidural abscess: a diagnostic challenge. Am Fam Physician 2002;65(7):1341–6.
22. Bulechek G, Butcher H, Dochterman J. Nursing interventions classification. 5th edtion. St. Louis, MO: Mosby; 2008. p. 430, 508–9, 532–3, 567–8, 709.
23. Saban K, Ghaly R. Spinal cervical infection: a case report and current update. J Neurosci Nurs 1998;30:105–15.

Ventriculitis of the Central Nervous System

Mary McKenna Guanci, MSN, RN, CNRN

KEYWORDS

- Intraventricular catheter • Cerebral spinal fluid • External ventricular drain • Shunt

KEY POINTS

- Ventriculitis commonly refers to an infection of the ventricular system.
- Ventriculitis has several possible causes.
- The signs and symptoms of ventriculitis include the triad of altered mental status, fever, and headache, as seen in the patient with meningitis.
- Intravenous antibiotics are usually chosen for management.

INTRODUCTION

Ventriculitis commonly refers to an infection of the ventricular system. The ventricular system consists of 2 lateral ventricles, a third and a fourth ventricle, and a series of aqueducts and foramina through which the cerebral spinal fluid (CSF) flows. CSF is produced by the choroid plexus in the ventricles and flows through the ventricular system of the brain and spinal cord. CSF flows through the foramen of Monro into the third ventricle through the sylvian aqueduct into the fourth ventricle. The foramen of Luschka and foramen of Magendie carry CSF into the subarachnoid space where it travels around the brain and spinal cord (**Fig. 1**).[1] CSF is clear and colorless with a protein content of 5 to 45 mg/dL and a glucose content of 50 to 75 mg/dL. The glucose content of the CSF makes it especially venerable to infectious processes. Arachnoid villi are responsible for reabsorption of CSF and, when CSF becomes infected, these arachnoid villi cannot reabsorb CSF at the necessary rate, resulting in hydrocephalus and possible increased intracranial pressure. The nurse caring for the patient at risk for ventriculitis must be aware of the cause, signs and symptoms, diagnosis, and treatment.

CAUSES

Ventriculitis may have several causes, including head trauma, brain abscess, infection including meningitis, pneumonia cranial or spinal cord surgery and placement and/or

Disclosures: None.
Neuroscience Intensive Care, Massachusetts General Hospital, 55 Fruit Street, Boston, MA 02474, USA
E-mail address: mguanci@partners.org

Crit Care Nurs Clin N Am 25 (2013) 399–406
http://dx.doi.org/10.1016/j.ccell.2013.04.005
0899-5885/13/$ – see front matter © 2013 Elsevier Inc. All rights reserved.

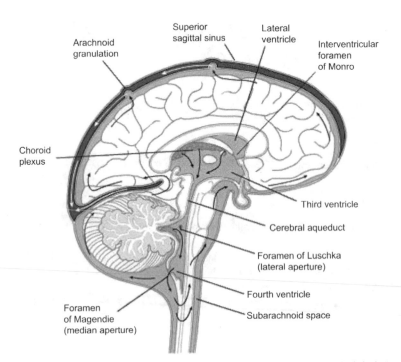

Fig. 1. CSF flow. (*Courtesy of* Rahul Gladwin, MD. *From* http://www.rahulgladwin.com/noteblog/miscellaneous/random-usmle-facts-volume-10-4.php; with permission.)

management of intracranial devices including ventricular shunts and catheters.[1,2] The number of possible causes and lack of data make it difficult to estimate the overall prevalence. Most available evidence comes from complication data after craniotomy and ventriculostomy. Ventricular catheter infection rates are estimated at 0% to 22%, with the average incidence less than 10%.[2] Ventricular shunt infections occur at a rate of 2.2% to 39%.[3] Meningitis from multiple causes occurs in 5 in 100,000 people per year in the United States.[4] There are no specific data about the number of these people who develop ventriculitis; however, bacterial meningitis often leads to ventriculitis. Bacterial meningitis and ventricular infection occurs in 1% to 2% of patients with traumatic brain injury with CSF leak. A fracture of the base of the skull increases this risk to 25%.[5]

SYMPTOMS

The signs and symptoms of ventriculitis include the triad of altered mental status, fever, and headache, as seen in the patient with meningitis. Irritability, limited eye up-gaze, and photophobia may also be present. In an intensive care, it may be difficult to assess the patient for these signs because of an already compromised level of consciousness and fever. The symptoms of hydrocephalus and increased intracranial pressure including pupillary change, motor weakness, and seizure should be considered in any assessment.

DIAGNOSTICS

Ventriculitis is not easily defined because of lack of research that might articulate the difference between infection and the contamination and colonization that may occur from placement and management of devices such as shunts and ventricular catheters. The US Center for Disease Control and Prevention (CDC) defines ventriculitis using symptoms and CSF findings (**Box 1**). Lozier and Sciacca[6] further described ventriculitis as having the characteristic clinical signs accompanied by fever, a low cerebral spinal glucose level, high CSF protein, and CSF pleocytosis. Comparisons of ventriculitis contamination and colonization are listed in **Box 1**.

Identifying the organism responsible using a CSF Gram stain and culture is important in determining the cause and in planning a treatment strategy. Culture results often require time and this diagnosis should be made rapidly because of the high-risk nature of the disease. CSF lactic acid levels including the presence of immunoglobulin G bands, CSF lactate, and lysozymes have been used to enhance early diagnosis. There are clinical situations that may interfere with the interpretation of any CSF testing results, such as hypoglycorrhachia (low CSF glucose). This inflammatory response is seen in subarachnoid hemorrhage or an injury in which blood in the brain is present. The clinicians should be aware that CSF alone may not be used to diagnose the disease. If the person has received antibiotics before the CSF sampling is obtained, absence of a positive culture is possible.

Coagulase-negative staphylococci, gram-negative bacilli, and *Staphylococcus aureus* are the most common species responsible for ventriculitis.[7] Different pathogens may be seen based on the possible cause. For example, *Streptococcus pneumoniae* and gram-negative rods are often seen in ventriculitis following head trauma. Gram-positive cocci and Acinetobacter are common findings in catheter-related ventriculitis. The growing problem of resistant strains of methicillin-resistant *S aureus* and coagulase-negative *Staphylococcus epidermidis* provides challenges in patient management. Sensitivity testing enables the clinician to target the appropriate antibiotic choice for the patient.

Imaging has been used in the diagnosis of ventriculitis, although it is more commonly used to evaluate the presence of hydrocephalus or increased intracranial pressure. (**Fig. 2**) shows a ventriculitis seen in the occipital horns of a patient after hemangioblastoma and external ventricular drain. Fukui[8] described the use of magnetic resonance imaging and computed tomography and concluded that the most frequent sign of radiographic ventriculitis was the appearance of debris in the CSF during diffusion-weighted imaging, periventricular hyperintense signaling, and ventricular ependymal enhancement.

TREATMENT

The management of ventriculitis is governed by the age of the patient, the cause of the infection, and the choice of the antibiotic based on CSF culture. The blood-brain barrier limits the use of antibiotics that may be chosen to treat a central nervous system infection. Intravenous antibiotics are chosen most often for management. Vancomycin is the drug of choice for treatment of staphylococci including *S aureus*, *S epidermidis*, or gram-negative bacilli. Linezolid in combination with a third-generation or fourth-generation cephalosporin such as cefepime has also been recommended, especially when the ventriculitis is caused by enterobacter and pseudomonas meningitis. There is evidence that *S pneumoniae*, and hemolytic streptococci respond to a third-generation cephalosporin with vancomycin or linezolid.[9] If ventriculitis is thought to be unresponsive to intravenous treatment or if considered to be more critical, intrathecal vancomycin can be administered using an intraventricular catheter (IVC) or an implanted device such as an Ommaya reservoir. Intraventricular administration of antibiotics is not recommended in neonates and was found to increase mortality 3-fold.[10]

Box 1
Diagnostic characteristics of ventriculitis

Adult:

1. Organism cultured from the CSF

2. Patient has at least 1 of the following signs or symptoms with no other recognized cause:

   a. Fever (38.8 C)

   b. Headache

   c. Stiff neck

   d. Meningeal sign

   e. Cranial nerve signs

   f. Irritability

3. One of the following CSF findings:

   a. Increased white cells, increased protein, and/or decreased glucose in CSF

   b. Organisms seen on Gram stain of CSF

   c. Organisms cultured from blood

   d. Positive antigen test of CSF, blood, or urine

   e. Diagnostic single-antibody titer (immunoglobulin [Ig] M) or 4-fold increase in paired sera (IgG) for pathogen

Infant 1 year old or less

1. Patient less than or equal to 1 year of age with at least 1 of the following signs or symptoms with no other recognized cause:

   a. Fever (38.8 C rectal)

   b. Hypothermia (37.8 C rectal)

   c. Apnea

   d. Bradycardia

   e. Stiff neck

   f. Meningeal signs

   g. Cranial nerve signs

   h. Irritability

2. Patient less than or equal to 1 year of age with at least 1 of the following:

   a. Positive CSF examination with increased white cells, increased protein, and/or decreased glucose

   b. Positive Gram stain of CSF

   c. Organisms cultured from blood

   d. Positive antigen test of CSF, blood, or urine

   e. Diagnostic single-antibody titer (IgM) or 4-fold increase in paired sera (IgG) for a pathogen

Adapted from O'Grady NP, Alexander M, Burns LA, et al. Guidelines for the prevention of intra-vascular catheter-related infections, 2011. Bethesda (MD): Centers for Disease Control and Prevention. Available at: http://www.cdc.gov/hicpac/pdf/guidelines/bsi-guidelines-2011.pdf.

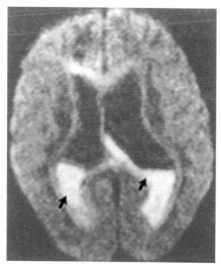

Fig. 2. Magnetic resonance imaging diffusion-weighted image of ventriculitis in occipital horns (*arrows*). (*From* Pezzullo JA, Tung GA, Mudigonda S, et al. Diffusion-weighted MR imaging of pyogenic ventriculitis. AJR Am J Roentgenol 2003;180:71–5; with permission.)

EXTERNAL VENTRICULAR DRAINS AND VENTRICULITIS

IVCs provide the care team with the ability to measure intracranial pressure, drain CSF into an external drainage system, sample CSF, or to instill medication into the ventricles. An IVC is inserted in the emergency department, intensive care unit, or in the operating room and may be managed in the intensive care unit or a neuroscience specialty acute care floor. The catheter is often placed in patients following head trauma to manage intracranial pressure, subarachnoid hemorrhage to manage hydrocephalus, or to manage CSF leaks after surgery. The infection rate of the catheter ranges from 0% to 49%, which may be attributed to insertion technique, maintenance of the system, and duration of insertion. Patency evaluation of the ventricular drainage system is an important factor. Problems that decrease flow of CSF into the drainage bag, such as kinks, blood, or particulate matter, may lead to neurologic change from increased intracranial pressure. One technique used to check patency of CSF flow is to briefly drop the ventricular drainage bag below the tragus or external auditory meatus and look for small CSF. The duration of the catheterization varies depending on the reason for use. There is controversy in the literature about the length of time a catheter is in place and the relationship to infection risk. Some studies support the catheter being left in place until it is no longer needed for therapy. Others suggest that routine reinsertion may be of benefit. The most recent study by Lyke[11] found that the duration of IVC use longer than 6 days and the existence of a previous IVC increased the risk of infection. The routine changing of an IVC is not recommended. Routine sampling of CSF is also not supported but should be included in a fever work-up for possible infection. There is evidence for the perioperative use of antibiotics to minimize the introduction of skin flora at the surgical site and perhaps into the CSF. Lozier and Sciacca[6] support the use of prophylactic antibiotics when weighed against the risk of ventriculitis. There is a concern that these prophylactic antibiotics increase the risk of infection from drug-resistant organisms. There are no guidance documents for how often the dressing change should occur. Guidance for dressing changes may be found using CDC guidelines for other invasive lines. A clear dressing provides direct visualization of the incision and allows monitoring of the wound bed. The recommendation is for change at least every 7 days or when needed. If the dressing does not allow visualization, then dressings are changed every 48 hours.[12] There is no difference in infection rate between transparent or adhesive dressings.[13] There is evidence that the use of drug impregnated may assist in reducing ventriculitis. Catheters impregnated with silver, rifampin, or clindamycin are available and are used in many hospitals for patients in whom the need for longer term ventriculostomy is anticipated.[14]

Collaborative guidelines for care of the patient with an IVC and ventricular drainage system should be available. The guideline should include recommendations for patient assessment, orders for height of drainage system, monitoring of intracranial pressure, and inspection of the catheter insertion site for a CSF leak. Maintenance of the IVC drainage system, including guidance for careful sampling of CSF by qualified staff, emptying the CSF collection bag, dressing changes, and continued documentation of date of catheter insertion, is also important. A discussion of the plan for the discontinuation of the IVC should occur during interdisciplinary rounds each day to ensure prompt removal.

LUMBAR DRAINS

A lumbar drain may also be used to drain CSF. The risk of ventriculitis is the same as for an external ventricular drain (EVD), although there are not enough prevalence data available in the literature. Scheihauer and colleagues[15] compared rates for IVC with rates for lumbar drain, and the risk factors for menigoventriculitis included lumbar drains, a previous menigoventriculitis, and presence of a neoplasm. The rate of lumbar drain infection was higher than that of IVC. Lumbar drain placement presents issues because of its location. The patient who is mobile may dislodge the dressing or tubing and requires education about risk. The nurse should check frequently to ensure patency and placement, and to ensure there is no CSF leak at the insertion site.

VENTRICULITIS AND SHUNT INFECTION

Ventricular shunts are used to divert CSF from the lateral ventricles to the peritoneum, atria, or pleural space. The presence of an implanted CSF device greatly increases ventriculitis risk. Children are thought to be at higher risk because of the length of time the shunt may be present and the immaturity of the immune system, but this has not been supported in the literature. A CSF leak caused by shunt integrity is thought to be responsible for the greatest risk.[16] Nurses should be alert to the signs of possible shunt infection, including fever, decreased level of consciousness, abdominal pain (if ventricular-peritoneal), and/or sepsis. Shunt malfunction occurs because infected CSF impedes drainage. Observing the patient for the signs and symptoms of increased intracranial pressure is also necessary. Recommended treatment of shunt infection includes removal of the infected appliance, placement of an IVC and external drainage device, and antibiotic therapy. The shunt is replaced once the patient is infection free and if it has been determined on reevaluation that continued assistance with ventricular drainage is needed.

NURSING MANAGEMENT OF VENTRICULITIS

Nurses have a pivotal role in the early identification and management of the patient with ventriculitis. General procedures for prevention of hospital-acquired infection, such as hand hygiene, should be enforced. Careful assessment of the patient for signs of neurologic change and advocating for rapid work-up of the febrile patient ensures comprehensive care. If the patient is having temperature regulated by a cooling device, changes reflecting possible temperature spikes should trigger an infection work-up including CSF if an intraventricular or lumbar drain catheter is present. The nurse is also in the position to promote best practice in the insertion, monitoring, and management of an IVC and drainage system if present. A safety assessment must be made in any confused or cognitively impaired patient to ensure the catheter remains is not removed accidentally. Monitoring patients after craniotomy or craniectomy for CSF leak, as well as patients with traumatic brain injury, helps with prompt detection and treatment. Advocating for quality initiatives in your facility promoting decreased or zero-tolerance ventriculitis rates raises awareness of patient risk and hospital performance. The literature provides examples of hospitals that have reduced ventricular catheter infection rates.[17] Family and patient education about the risks associated with ventriculitis, explanation of any ventricular devices, signs and symptoms of infection, and the plan of care are important to the promotion of patient-centered/family-centered care.

More ventriculitis research is needed to help identify which patients are at highest risk and which treatment regimes are the most effective. Data collection for tracking rates of infection is hampered by the lack of consensus for standard measurement. Some research supports reporting infection per catheter day, whereas some gives a percentage of total infections. Ventriculitis is currently not reported in the hospital-acquired infection database but, given the current trends and the incidence of infection related to implantable devices, it seems to be a natural progression. So-called superbugs, or antibiotic-resistant microbes, will challenge clinical teams to adequately treat patients. Nursing will play a pivotal role in future research and the development of strategies to prevent an infection of the ventricular system.

REFERENCES

1. Bader M, Littlejohns L. Core curriculum of neuroscience nursing. Chicago IL: American Association of Neuroscience Nursing; 2008. p. 34–5.
2. Agrawal A, Cincu R. Current concepts and approach to ventriculitis. Infect Dis Clin Pract 2008;6(2):100–4.
3. Sacar S. A retrospective study of central nervous system shunt infections diagnosed in a university hospital during a 4-year period. BMC Infect Dis 2006; 6(43):1–5.
4. VanDemark M. Infectious and autoimmune processes. In: Bader MK, Littlejohns L, editors. Core curriculum of neuroscience nurses. Chicago IL: American Association of Neuroscience Nurses. Chapter 19. 2008. p. 605–51.
5. Beer R. Infectious intracranial complications in the neuro-ICU patient population. Curr Opin Crit Care 2010;16:117–22.
6. Lozier A, Sciacca R. Ventriculostomy-related infection; critical review of the literature. Neurosurgery 2002;51(1):170–81.
7. Celik S. Nosocomial infections in neurosurgery intensive care units. J Clin Nurs 2004;13:741–7.
8. Fukui M, Williams R. Am J Neuroradiol 2001;22:1510–6.
9. Cook AM, Ramsey CN, Martin CA, et al. Linezolid for the treatment of a heteroresistant *Staphylococcus aureus* shunt infection. Pediatr Neurosurg 2005;41: 102–4.

10. Shah S. Intraventricular antibiotics for bacterial meningitis in neonates. Cochran Collaboration. New Jersey: Wiley; 2012.

11. Lyke K, Obasanjo O. Clinical Infectious Diseases 2001;33:2028–33.

12. CDC Guidelines. Available at: http://www.cdc.gov/hicpac/pdf/guidelines/bsi-guidelines-2011.pdf. Accessed December 2012.

13. Shultz M. Bacterial ventriculitis and duration of ventriculostomy catheter insertion. J Neurosci Nurs 1993;25(3):158–64.

14. Lemcke J, Depner F. The impact of silver nanoparticle-coated and antibiotic-impregnated external ventricular drainage catheters on the risk of infection: a clinical comparison of 95 patients. Acta Neurochir Suppl 2012;114:347–50.

15. Scheithauer S, Bürgel U, Bickenbach J, et al. External ventricular and lumbar drainage-associated meningoventriculitis: prospective analysis of time-dependent infection rates and risk factor analysis. Infection 2010;38:205–9.

16. Tamburrini G. Diagnosis and management of shunt complications in the treatment of childhood hydrocephalus. World Federation of Neurosurgery. Available at: www.wfns.org/pages/read_the_reviews/97.php?rid=5. Accessed December 2012.

17. Hill M. A multidisciplinary approach to end external ventricular drain infections in the neurocritical care unit. J Neurosci Nurs 2012;44(4):188–93.

Index

Note: Page numbers of article titles are in **boldface** type.

A

Abcess(es), brain, **381–388**
  spinal epidural, **389–397**
Acute bacterial meningitis, **351–361**
  clinical presentation of, meningeal signs, in adults, 353
    in neonates and infants, 353
    symptoms in, 353
  defined, 351–352
  diagnosis of, algorithm for, 355
    CSF analysis in, 354–355
    differentiation of bacterial *vs.* aseptic meningitis in, 355
    head CT in, 354–355
    lumbar puncture in, 354
  epidemiology of, causative pathogens in, 352
    populations at risk for, 352
  incidence of, 352
  nursing management of, fluid management in, 357
    neurologic monitoring in, 457
    supportive care in, 357
  outcome of, indicators of poor prognosis, 358–359
    neurologic sequelae, 358
    systemic complications, 358
  pathophysiology of, bacteremia from systemic infection in, 352–353
    cerebral damage in, 353
    nasopharyngeal colonization in, 352
  prevention of, chemoprophylaxis for, 357–358
    vaccinations for, 358
  treatment of, adjunctive corticosteroids in, 356–357
    empiric antimicrobial therapy in, 356
Adenovirus, in viral meningitis, 369
Arboviral encephalitis, blood-sucking vector in, 374
  common causes of, 374
  prevention of, 374

B

Brain abcess, **381–388**
  clinical manifestations of, focal neurologic deficits, 383
    symptoms, 383
  diagnosis of, CT with contrast in, 383–384
    gadolinium-enhanced MRI in, 384
    laboratory specimens in, 384

Crit Care Nurs Clin N Am 25 (2013) 407–410
http://dx.doi.org/10.1016/S0899-5885(13)00061-0
0899-5885/13/$ – see front matter © 2013 Elsevier Inc. All rights reserved.

ccnursing.theclinics.com

Brain (*continued*)
  nursing considerations, neurologic examination and serial assessment in, 385–386
    prevention of nosocomial infection, 386
  outcomes, traditional and modern, 381
  pathogenesis of, common organisms in, 382
    direct spread in, 382
    hematogenous seeding and spread in, 382–383
  pathophysiology of, sites of, 382
  prognosis for, factors in, 381–382
  treatment of, antibiotics in, 384–385
    needle aspiraton of, 384
    surgical drainage and excision in, 384

C

Cerebrospinal fluid, characterization of, 399–400
Coxsackie virus, in viral meningitis, 366

E

Echoviruses, in viral meningitis, 367
Encephalitis. See *Viral encephalitis.*
Enteroviruses, in viral meningitis, 366

H

Herpes simplex virus, in viral encephalitis, CSF fluid in, 373
    CT findings in, 374
    HSV-2 sexual contact spread of, 373
    HSV-1 transmission in, 373
    outcome of, 374
    symptoms of, 373
Herpes virus-1 (HSV-1), in viral meningitis, 367–368
Herpes virus-2 (HSV-2), in viral meningitis, 368

L

Lymphocytic choriomeningitis, in viral meningitis, 369

M

Meningitis, bacterial, **351–361**
  viral, **363–369**
Mollaret meningitis, 368
Mosquito-borne encephalitis, Eastern equine encephalitis, 374–375
  La Crosse encephalitis, in children, 375
    in woodland animals, 376
  St. Louis encephalitis, 376
  Venezuelan equine encephalitis, 375
  Western equine encephalitis, 375
  West Nile virus, 376–377
Mumps CNS syndromes, in viral meningitis, 368

P

Paramyxovirus, in viral meningitis, 368
Poliovirus, in viral meningitis, 367

R

Rabies, from bite of infected animal, 378
    2010 cases in U.S., 377–378
    forms of, dumb/paralytic, 378
        furious, 378
    incubation period for, 378
    postexposure prophylaxis, 378–379

S

Spinal epidural abscess (SEA), nursing care in, neurologic assessments, 393–394
Spinal epidural abscess (SEA), **389–397**
    comorbidities in, 390
    diagnosis of, clinical presentation in, 390–391
        CT with myelography, 391
        imaging in, gadolinium-enhanced MRI, 391
        laboratory testing in, 390–391
        microbiological studies in, 391
    epidemiology of, age and, 390
        predisposing conditions, 389
        rising incidence in, 389
    nursing care in, infection and, 395
        pain management, 393–395
        patient education, 395
        positioning and mobility, 395
        potential interventions, 393–394
        rehabilitation programs and, 395
        self-management strategies, 395
    outcomes, with urgent surgery *vs.* nonoperative approach, 393
    predisposing conditions for, 390
    from Staphylococcus aureus, 389
    surgical consult in, 391–392
    treatment of, conservative, 393
        CT-guided needle aspiration, 392
        pharmacologic, 392
        surgical, decompressive, 392
            hemi-laminectomy, 392

V

Varicella zoster virus, in viral meningitis, 368
Ventriculitis, causes of, 399–400
    of central nervous system, **399–406**
    cerebrospinal fluid and, 399
    definition of, 399
    diagnostics in, 400–402

Ventriculitis (*continued*)

    imaging, 401, 403

    sensitivity testing of CSF, 401

   intraventricular drainage system and, care of, 404

    dressing changes and, 403–404

    prophylactic antibiotics and, 403

   lumbar drains and, 404

   nursing management of, family and patient education in, 405

    general procedures, 404–405

    patient assessments in, 405

   and shunt infection, 404

   symptoms of, 400

   treatment of, intravenous antibiotics in, 401

Viral encephalitis, **369–379**

   causes of, 373–379

   clinical manifestations of, 371

   diagnosis of, CSF analysis in, 371–372

    EEG in, 372

    laboratory testing, 371

    neuroimaging in, 371

   epidemiology of, characteristics and laboratory diagnosis of, 369–371

    direct injection into bloodstream, 369

    person-to-person transmission in, 369

   etiology of, 371

   grouping and mode of transmission of, 371

   treatment of, acyclovir for, 372

    algorithm for, 372

    supportive care in, 372

   vaccines for, 373

Viral meningitis, 363, **363–369**

   causes of, 366–369

   clinical manifestations of, 365

   diagnosis of, CSF analysis in, 365

    data for, 366

    lumbar puncture in, 365

    risk factors for, 366

   epidemiology of, viruses in, 364–365

   etiology of, viruses in, 365

   viruses in neurologic disease, 364

   vs. aseptic meningitis, 363

W

West Nile virus infection, acute *vs.* asymptomatic illness, 377

   characterization of, 377

   dementia and paralysis following, 377

   modes of transmission, 377

   mosquito-borne, 376–377

   serologic diagnosis of, 377

HEALTHCARE LIBRARY
52 GOWER STREET
LONDON WC1E 6EB
03-447-097
BLOOMSBURY LIBRARY

BLOOMSBURY
HEALTHCARE LIBRARY
52 GOWER STREET
LONDON WC1E 6EB
03-447-9097